CW00953177

FOOD
COMBINING
MADE EASY

Herbert Shelton

Published by:
BOOK PUBLISHING COMPANY
SUMMERTOWN, TENNESSEE

Library of Congress Cataloging-in-Publication Data

Shelton, Herbert M. (Herbert McGolphin), 1895-1985.
 Food combining made easy / by Herbert M. Shelton.
   p. cm.
 Originally published: San Antonio, Tex. : Willow Pub., [c1982].
 ISBN 978-1-57067-260-6 (pbk.)
 1. Food combining. 2. Nutrition. I. Title.
 RA784.S523 2012
 613.2--dc23
                           2011040943

Book Publishing Company
P.O. Box 99
Summertown, TN 38483
888-260-8458
bookpubco.com

ISBN 13: 978-1-57067-260-6

Printed on recycled paper

Book Publishing Company is a member of Green Press Initiative. We chose to print this title on paper with 30% post consumer recycled content, processed without chlorine, which saved the following natural resources:

- 10 trees
- 293 pounds of solid waste
- 4,621 gallons of water
- 1,025 pounds of greenhouse gases
- 4 million BTU of energy

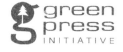

For more information on Green Press Initiative, visit www.greenpressinitiative.org. Environmental impact estimates were made using the Environmental Defense Fund Paper Calculator. For more information visit www.papercalculator.org.

CONTENTS

FOREWORD

Herbert Shelton was a nutritional pioneer in the early twentieth century and founder of the natural hygiene movement. He inspired scores of individuals, including Mahatma Gandhi and George Bernard Shaw, to adopt the principles of fasting and the use of raw, plant-based diets.

In Shelton's time, the public was not as familiar or comfortable with the idea of replacing meat and fish with plant proteins as we are today. In earlier editions of *Food Combining Made Easy*, he reached out to a broad base of readers by including recommendations for how to incorporate foods he didn't normally espouse in a daily diet.

Currently, plant-based diets are not only popular, they are acknowledged by many in the scientific community as being the ideal choice for health and longevity. We feel Shelton would be pleased at this development. In this current edition of the book, we've chosen to remove recommendations for the use of meat and fish in the diet to more closely reflect Shelton's personal practices and recommendations.

We have retained any deleted original text in the form of notes, which are indicated by reference numbers in the body of the book and found in the reference section at the back.

Cynthia Holzapfel
Managing Editor
Book Publishing Company

INTRODUCTION

A few years ago I sat with a group in the home of a friend and viewed a television program. On one of the commercials a cereal bowl was placed before us on the viewing screen. Before our eyes a huckster poured the bowl full of a popular breakfast food. Into this, he dumped two heaping teaspoonfuls of white sugar. Over this he sliced a banana and poured onto the mixture he had created, a handful of raisins. Finally, he poured over the whole mixture a liberal quantity of milk or cream, which was sure to have been pasteurized. As he demonstrated the preparation of the breakfast dish, he kept up a running fire of words intended to convince the television audience that the mixture of food he had put together was both tasty and nutritious.

When he had finished, one of the young women in our group said: "When I eat a meal like that, I always have heartburn." To this I remarked: "You and several million other people." No digestive system known to man is adapted to the digestion of such a meal.

No animal in nature ever eats such a haphazard commingling of heterogeniety. It does not speak well for human intelligence that millions of men, women and children, continue to eat such meals day after day and take drugs to palliate the resulting discomforts.

Many millions of dollars are spent every year for antacids and other drugs to *relieve* the gastric distress that is almost inevitable after a meal of this kind. To name a few popular drugs, most of which contain bicarbonate of soda (baking soda), there are Alka·Seltzer, Tums, Bellans, Pepto·Bismol, Rolaids, Di-Gel, etc. In addition to these patent nostrums, many people still use the old stand by of yesteryear, sodium bicarbonate. Others use Milk of Magnesia. These drugs, while producing troubles of their own, provide the foolish with temporary relief from the discomforts of indigestion.

In the face of all the unnecessary suffering that millions undergo daily and the tremendous expense of the *relief* they seek, there are still many who decry the effort to obviate all their suffering by the simple process of eating properly combined meals.

There is an old adage, which says: "The proof of the pudding is in the eating thereof." What we say about food combining is of such a character that the ordinary untechnically trained man and woman may make it for himself. It does not require an expensive laboratory for testing, but may be done at home by the simple plan of eating meals combined according to the rules contained in our literature and note the results. The results obtained may then be compared with the results of the previous haphazard eating.

Not long since, one of my distributors received a letter from a woman in Pennsylvania, to whom he sold a copy of "Food Combining Made Easy." He sent me a Xeroxed copy of the letter. I give relevant portions of the letter herewith: "Writing fan mail letters is not one of my many bad habits, but this is more than a fan letter. It is a letter of appreciation, gratitude and thanks.

"What a fortunate day it was for me when I received your literature and sent for the booklet 'Food Combining Made Easy' by H. M. Shelton.

"For years I suffered with indigestion, gas, bloating and real discomfort and pain. Now I am trying to combine food properly and the indigestion and discomfort has left. No more gas, bloating, Tums, Rolaids, soda or Alka-Seltzer.

"Why do not more people try this simple method? I'm sure it is because they do not know."

I have received numerous letters like the foregoing. Many have talked to me personally and testified to the same fact. Great numbers of them have asserted that they found relief with the first properly combined meal. Only recently a man, telling me of his experiences, stated that his whole family had been freed of their after-meal discomfort by eating properly combined meals. He and his family had also found that they can get along without drugs. Many more have told me how their so-called allergies to various foods came to an end when they learned to combine their foods properly.

The human digestive tract was not designed by nature to digest complex meals. Seven course meals and twenty-one course dinners were not in nature's plan when she designed the human digestive tract. The man who sits down to a dining table that is burdened with a great variety of foods and eats everything from "soup to nuts," is sure to suffer with indigestion. If he makes a habit of eating complex meals and disregarding his enzymic limitations, as is customary, his abdominal distress will be chronic. He is likely to carry a supply of pills with him wherever he goes. Indeed, the practice of carrying pills in one's vest pocket or in one's purse is encouraged by the makers of pills. It seems that it is more important for one to have at hand a means of fictional relief than to learn to eat sensibly and thus avoid the apparent need for the *relief*. Perhaps it is important to enrich the drug manufacturers, even at the expense of one's own health.[1]

From medical sources, as well as from the camp-followers of medicine in the other schools of so-called healing, and the dietetic camp-followers of Allopathy, certain objections are made to the practice of avoiding certain food combinations and eating others. These objections are all based on the assumption that the human stomach is equipped to easily and efficiently digest any and all possible combinations of foods that may be introduced into it. Very little special attention will be devoted to meeting these objections, as the facts presented in this little book constitute sufficient reply to the objections.

More than sixty years spent in feeding and caring for the young and the old, the well and the sick, male and female, rich and poor, educated and ignorant, more than fifty years of this spent in institutional practice, the balance in office practice, certainly entitle me to speak with some degree of authority of this subject. I have spent more than sixty years in the study of dietetics, and I have directed the care and feeding of many thousands of people. I submit to the intelligent reader the thought that such an experience better qualifies me to speak upon the subject that forms the text of this little book than an equal time devoted to drugging the sick. Few medical men make a study of dietetics and still fewer of them make any extensive use of it in their care of their patients. Their usual advice to their patients is to "eat whatever agrees with you."

It is not asserted in this book that any program of diet, nor any program of food combining, will cure disease. I do not believe in cures. I assert and am ready to prove, that in all cases of sickness, where organic damage is not too great for vital redemption, when cause is removed the forces and processes of life, working with the normal materials of life, will restore health and integrity. Food is but one of the normal materials of life.

As an indispensable basis of the work of the *Hygienist,* we must endeavor to secure to the health seeker the full benefit of all the Hygienic means, in their entire plenitude, for only thus can the health seeker be given a fair chance of recovery. The intelligent reader should have no difficulty in understanding that Hygienic care is the only rational and radical care that has ever been administered to the sick in any age of the world at any place. The time must come when all forms of disease will be "treated" on the broad and infallible basis of Hygienic principles. When true principles are discovered, they are found to apply, not to one or two diseases only, nor to but one class of diseases, but all diseases whatsoever. The same fundamental principles will apply throughout the whole catalogue of diseases. Even in those cases where surgery can be of value, Hygienic care should always be employed as the groundwork for the surgery.

Why give attention to the combinations of food eaten? Why not combine our foods indiscriminately and eat haphazardly? Why give thought and attention to such matters? Do animals follow rules of food combining?

The answers to these questions are simple. Let us start with the last question. Animals eat very simply and do very little combining. Certainly the meat eating animal consumes no carbohydrates with his proteins. He does not take acids with his proteins. The deer grazing in the forest combines his foods very little. The squirrel, eating nuts, is likely to eat his fill of nuts and take no other food with these. Birds have been observed to eat insects at one time of day, seeds at another. No animal in a state of nature has the great variety of different foods spread before it at a meal that civilized man has. Primitive man had no such great variety of foods at a meal. He, too, ate simply, as do the animals.

As will be seen later, the digestive enzymes of the human digestive tract have certain well defined limitations and when we eat in such a manner as .to over-ride these limitations, we run into digestive troubles. Proper food combining is merely a sane way of respecting our enzymic limitations. We combine our foods properly and do not eat haphazardly and indiscriminately, because, by so doing, we assure better and more efficient digestion of our foods.

We derive no value from foods that are not digested. To eat and have the food spoil in the digestive tract is to waste the food. It is worse than this, as the spoiling of foods results in the production of poisons which are injurious. Proper food combining, therefore, not only assures better nutrition, as a consequence of better digestion of our foods, but it provides for a protection against poisoning.

An amazing number of food allergies clear up completely when supposedly allergic individuals learn to eat their foods in digestible combinations. What they suffer from is not allergy, as this is at present understood, but indigestion. Allergy is a term applied to protein poisoning. Indigestion results in putrefactive poisoning, which is also a form of protein poisoning. Normal digestion delivers nutrients, not poisons to the blood stream. Fully digested proteins are not poisonous substances.

With knowledge based on wide experience, then, I offer this little book to the intelligent reader, in the hope that he will make full use of its information to the end that he may enjoy better health and a longer and more abundant life. To the doubter I say only: Give it a trial and convince yourself. It has truly been said that condemnation without investigation is a bar to all knowledge. Do not cut yourself off from further knowledge and from better health by condemning, without a fair test, the simple rules that are presented in this little book.

FOODSTUFFS CLASSIFIED

F ood is that material which can be incorporated into and become a part of the cells and fluids of the body. Non-useful materials, such as drugs, are all poisonous. To be a true food, the substance eaten must not contain useless or harmful ingredients. For example, tobacco, which is a plant, contains proteins, carbohydrates, minerals, vitamins and water. As such, it should be a food. But, in addition to these materials, it also contains considerable quantities of poisons, one of these, one of the most virulent poisons known to science. Tobacco, therefore, is not a food.

Foodstuffs as we get them from the garden and orchard or from the food store, or in the raw state, are composed of water and a few organic compounds known as proteins, carbohydrates (sugars, starches, pentosans), fats (oils), mineral salts and vitamins. They commonly possess more or less of non-usable or indigestible matter - waste.

Foods as we get them from the garden and orchard or purchase them from the food store are the raw materials of nutrition. They vary widely in character and quality, hence, for convenience, are classified according to their composition and sources of origin. The following classifications of foods will guide the reader in his combinations.

PROTEINS
Protein foods are those that contain a high percentage of protein in their makeup. Chief among these are the following:

Nuts	All flesh foods (*Except fat*)
All cereals	Cheese
Dry beans	Olives
Dry peas	Avocados
Soy beans	Milk *(low protein)*
Peanuts	

STARCHES

The carbohydrates are the starches and sugars. I have broken these up into three distinct groups in the following classification - starches, sugars, syrups, and sweet fruits.

STARCHES

All cereals	Hubbard squash
Dry beans *(except Soy beans)*	Banana squash
Dry peas	Pumpkin
Potatoes *(all kinds)*	Caladium root
Chestnuts	Jerusalem artichokes
Peanuts	

MILDLY STARCHY

Cauliflower	Rutabaga
Beets	Salsify
Carrots	

SYRUPS AND SUGARS

Brown sugar	Maple syrup
White sugar	Cane syrup
Milk sugar	Honey

SWEET FRUITS

Banana	Persimmon
Date	Mangoes
Fig	Cherimoya
Raisin	Papaya
Thompson & Muscat grape	Cherry
Prune	Sun-dried pear

FATS

The fats are all fats and oils, as follow:

Olive Oil	Nut Oils
Soy Oil	Corn Oils
Sunflower Seed Oil	Tallow

Sesame Oil	Most Nuts
Butter substitutes	Fat meats
Pecans	Lard
Butter	Cotton Seed Oil
Cream	Avocados

ACID FRUITS

Most of the acids eaten as foods are acid fruits. Chief among these are:

Orange	Lime
Grapefruit	Sour Apple
Pineapple	Sour Grape
Pomegranate	Sour Peach
Tomato	Sour Plum
Lemon	

SUB-ACID FRUITS

The sub-acid fruits are as follow:

Fresh fig	Sweet Apple
Pear	Apricot
Sweet cherry	Huckleberry
Sweet Peach	Sweet Plum

NON-STARCHY AND GREEN VEGETABLES

Into this classification fall all succulent vegetables without regard for their color, whether green, red, yellow, or white, etc. Chief among these are:

Lettuce	Collards
Celery	Spinach
Endive *(French)*	Chard
Chicory	Okra
Cabbage	Cucumber
Cauliflower	Sorrel
Broccoli	Asparagus
Brussel Sprouts	

Cow-slip
Chinese Cabbage
Chive
Mustard
Dock *(sour)*
Turnip
Kale
Mulliein

Rape
Green Corn
Eggplant
Kohlrabi
Cardoon
Radish
Parsley

Rhubard
Watercress
Onions
Scallions
Leeks
Garlic
Zuccini

Escarole
Beet tops (greens)
Turnip tops (greens)
Bamboo sprouts
Broccoli-de-Rappe
Dandelion
Sweet Pepper

MELONS

Water melon
Musk melon
Honey dew
Honey balls
Casaba
Cantaloupe

Pie melon
Banana melon
Crenshaw melon
Christmas melon
Persian melon
Nutmeg melon

DIGESTION OF FOODS

Foodstuffs, as we eat them constitute the raw materials of nutrition. As proteins, carbohydrates and fats, they are not usable by the body. They must first undergo a disintegrating, refining and standardizing process (more properly a series of processes) to which the term digestion has been given. Although this process of digestion is partly mechanical, as in the chewing, swallowing and" churning" of food, the physiology of digestion is very largely a study of the chemical changes foods undergo in their passage through the alimentary canal. For our present purposes, we need give but little attention to intestinal digestion, but will concentrate upon mouth and stomach digestion.

The changes through which foods go in the processes of digestion are effected by a group of agencies known as enzymes or unorganized ferments. Due to the fact that the conditions under which these enzymes can act are sharply defined, it becomes necessary to give heed to the simple rules of correct food combining that have been carefully worked out on a basis of the chemistry of digestion. Long and patient effort on the part of many physiologists in many parts of the world have brought to light a host of facts concerning enzymic limitations, but, unfortunately, these same physiologists have attempted to slur over their importance and to supply us with fictional reasons why we should continue to eat and drink in the conventionally haphazard manner. They have rejected every effort to make a practical application of the great fund of vital knowledge their painstaking labors have provided. Not so the *Natural Hygienists*. We seek to base our rules of life upon the principles of biology and physiology.

Let us briefly consider *enzymes* in general before we go on to a study of the enzymes of the mouth and stomach. An *enzyme* may be appropriately defined as a physiological *catalyst*. In the study of chemistry it was soon found that many substances that do not normally combine when brought into contact with each other, may be made to do so by a third substance when it is brought into contact with them. This third substance does not in any way enter into the combination, or share in the reaction, its mere presence seems to bring about the combination and reaction. Such a substance or agent is called a *catalyst* -the process is called *catalsis*.

Plants and animals manufacture soluble catalytic substances, colloidal in nature and but little resistant to heat, which they employ in the many processes of splitting up of compounds and the making of new ones within themselves. To these substances the term *enzyme* has been applied. Many *enzymes* are known, all of them, apparently, of protein character. The only ones that need interest us here are those involved in the digestion of foodstuffs. These are involved in the reduction of complex food substances to simpler compounds that are acceptable to the bloodstream and usable by the cells of the body in the production of new cell -substance.

As the action of enzymes in the digestion of foodstuffs closely resembles fermentation, these substances were formerly referred to as ferments. Fermentation, however, is accomplished by organized ferments - bacteria. The products of fermentation are not identical with the products of enzymic disintegration of foodstuffs and are not suitable as nutritive materials. Rather, they are poisonous. Putrefaction, also the result of bacterial action, also gives rise to poisons, some of them very virulent, rather than to nutritive materials. Each enzyme is specific in its action. This is to say, it acts only upon one class of food substance. The enzymes that act upon carbohydrates do not and cannot act upon proteins nor upon salts nor fats. They are even more specific than this would indicate. For example, in the digestion of closely related substances, such as the disaccharides (complex sugars), the enzyme that acts upon maltose is not capable of acting upon lactose. Each sugar seems to require its own specific enzyme. The physiologist, Howell, tells us that there is no clear proof that any single enzyme can produce more than one kind of ferment action.

This specific action of enzymes is of importance, as there are various stages in the digestion of foodstuffs, each stage requiring the action of a different enzyme, and the various enzymes being capable of performing their work only if the preceding work has been properly performed by the enzymes that also precede. If *pepsin,* for example, has not converted proteins into peptones, the enzymes that convert peptones into amino acids will not be able to act upon the proteins.

The substance upon which an enzyme acts is called a *substrate.* Thus starch is the substrate of *ptyalin.* Dr. N. Phillip Norman, formerly instructor in gastro·enterology, New York Polyclinic Medical School and Hospital, New York City, says: "In studying the action of different enzymes, one is struck by Emil Fischer's statement that there must be a special key to each lock. The ferment being the lock and its substrate the key, and if the key does not fit exactly in the lock, no reaction is possible. In view of this fact, is it not logical to believe the admixture of different types of carbohydrates and fats and proteins in the same meal to be distinctly injurious to the digestive cells? If, since it is true that similar, but not identical locks are produced by the same type of cells, it is logical to believe that this admixture taxes the physiological functions of these cells to their limit." Fischer, who was a renowned physiologist, suggested that the specificity of the various enzymes is related to the structure of substances acted upon. Each enzyme is apparently adapted to or fitted to a certain definite structure.

Digestion commences in the mouth. All foods are broken up into smaller particles by the process of chewing, and they are thoroughly saturated with saliva. Of the chemical part of digestion, only starch digestion begins in the mouth. The saliva of the mouth, which is normally an alkaline fluid, contains an enzyme called *ptyalin,* which acts upon starch, breaking this down into maltose, a complex sugar, which is further acted upon in the intestine by *maltase* and converted into the simple sugar *dextrose.* The action of ptyalin upon starch is preparatory, as maltase cannot act upon starch. *Amylase,* the starch-splitting enzyme of the pancreatic secretion, is said to act upon starch much as does *ptyalin,* so that starch that escapes digestion in the mouth and stomach may be split into maltose and achroodextrine, providing, of course, that it has not undergone fermentation before it reaches the intestine.

Ptyalin is destroyed by a mild acid and also by a strong alkaline reaction. It can act only in an alkaline medium and this must not be strongly alkaline. It is this limitation of the enzyme that renders important the manner in which we mix our starches, for if they are mixed with foods that are acid or that provide for an acid secretion in the stomach, the action of the *ptyalin* is brought to an end. We will learn more of this later.

Stomach, or gastric juice ranges all the way from nearly neutral in reaction to strongly acid, depending upon the character of the food eaten. It contains two enzymes - *pepsin,* which acts upon proteins; *lipase,* which has slight action upon fats. The only one of these enzymes that needs concern us here is pepsin. Pepsin is capable of initiating digestion in all kinds of proteins. This is important, as it seems to be the only enzyme with such power. Different protein splitting enzymes act upon the different stages of protein digestion. It is possible that none of them can act upon protein in stages preceding the stage for which they are specifically adapted. For example, *erepsin,* found in the intestinal juice and in the pancreatic juice, does not act upon complex proteins, but only upon peptids and polypeptids, reducing these to amino-acids. Without the prior action of pepsin in reducing the proteins to peptids, the erepsin would not act upon the protein food. Pepsin acts only in an acid medium and is destroyed by an alkali. Low temperature, as when iced drinks are taken, retards and even suspends the action of pepsin. Alcohol precipitates this enzyme.

Just as the sight, odor or thought of food may occasion a flow of saliva. a "watering of the mouth," so these same factors may cause a flow of gastric juice, that is a "watering of the stomach." The taste of food, however, is most important in occasioning a flow of saliva. The physiologist. Carlson, failed in repeated efforts to occasion a flow of gastric juice by having his subjects chew on different substances, or by irritating the nerve-endings in the mouth by substances other than those directly related to food. In other words, there is no secretory action when the substances taken into the mouth cannot be digested. There is selective action on the part of the body and. as will be seen later, there are different kinds of action for different kinds of foods.

In his experiments in studying the "conditioned reflex," Pavlov noted that it is not necessary to take the food into the mouth in order to occasion a flow of gastric juice. The mere teasing of a dog with savory food will serve. He found that even the noises or some other action associated with feeding time, will occasion a flow of secretion.

It is necessary that we devote a few paragraphs to a brief study of the body's ability to adapt its secretions to the different kinds of foodstuffs that are consumed. Later, we will discuss the limitations of this power. McLeod's *Physiology in* Modern *Medicine* says: The observations of Pavlov on the responses of gastric pouches of dogs to meat, bread, and milk have been widely quoted. They are interesting because they constitute evidence that the operation of the gastric secretory mechanism is not without some power of adaptation to the materials to be digested."

This adaptation is made possible by reason of the fact that the gastric secretions are the products of about five million microscopic glands embedded in the walls of the stomach, various of which secrete different parts of the gastric juice. The varying amounts and proportions of the various elements that enter into the composition of the gastric juice give a juice of varying characters and adapted to the digestion of different kinds of foodstuffs. Thus the juice may be almost neutral in reaction, it may be weakly acid or strongly acid. There may be more or less pepsin according to need. There is also the factor of timing. The character of the juice may be very different at one stage of digestion from what it is at another, as the varying requirements of a food are met.

A similar adaptation of saliva to different foods and digestive requirements is seen to occur. For example weak acids occasion a copious flow of saliva, while weak alkalis occasion no salivary secretion. Disagreeable and noxious substances also occasion salivary secretion, in this instance, to flush away the offending material. It is noted by physiologists that with at least two different types of glands in the mouth able to function, a considerable range of variation is possible with reference to the character of the mixed secretion finally discharged.

An excellent example of this ability of the body to modify and adapt its secretions to the varying needs of various kinds of foods is supplied us by the dog. Feed him flesh and there is a secretion of thick viscous saliva, chiefly from the submaxillary gland. Feed him dried and pulverized flesh and a very copious and watery secretion will be poured out upon it, coming from the parotid gland. The mucous secretion poured out upon flesh serves to lubricate the bolus of food and thus facilitate swallowing. The thin, watery secretion, on the other hand, poured out upon the dry powder, washes the powder from the mouth. Thus, it is seen that the kind of juice poured out is determined by the purpose it must serve.

As was previously noted, ptyalin has no action upon sugar. When sugar is eaten there is a copious flow of saliva, but it contains no ptyalin. If soaked starches are eaten, no saliva is poured out upon these. Ptyalin is not poured out upon flesh or fat. These evidences of adaptation are but a few of the many that could be given. It seems probable that a wider range of adaptation is possible in gastric than in salivary secretion. These things are not without their significance to the person who is desirous of eating in a manner to assure most efficient digestion, although it is the custom of physiologists to gloss over or minimize them. We shall have occasion to refer to these matters in greater detail in subsequent chapters.

There are reasons for believing that man, like the lower animals, once instinctively avoided wrong combinations of foods, and there are remnants of the old instinctive practices still extant. But having kindled the torches of intellect upon the ruins of instinct, man is compelled to seek out his way in a bewildering maze of forces and circumstances by the fool's method of trial and error. At least this is so until he has gained sufficient knowledge and a grasp of proved principles to enable him to govern his conduct in the light of principles and knowledge. Instead, then, of ignoring the great mass of laboriously accumulated physiological knowledge relating to the digestion of our foodstuffs, or glossing over them as is the practice of the professional physiologists, it behooves us, as intelligent beings, to make full and proper use of such knowledge. If the physiology of digestion can lead us to eating practices that insure better digestion, hence better nutrition, only the foolish will disregard its immense value to us, both in health and in disease.

RIGHT AND WRONG COMBINATIONS

To make fully clear what combinations of foodstuffs override our enzymic limitations it will be necessary to consider, one by one, the possible combinations and briefly discuss these in their relations to the facts of digestion which we learned in the previous chapter. Such a study should prove both interesting and instructive to the intelligent reader.

ACID-STARCH COMBINATIONS

In the last chapter we learned that a weak acid will destroy the ptyalin of the saliva. With the destruction of the ptyalin starch digestion must come to a halt. The physiologist Stiles says: "If the mixed food is quite acid at the outset, it is hard to see how there can be any hydrolysis (enzymic digestion of starch) brought about by the saliva. Yet we constantly eat acid fruits before our breakfast cereal and notice no ill effects. Starch which escapes digestion at this stage is destined to be acted upon by the pancreatic juice, and the final result may be entirely satisfactory. Still it is reasonable to assume that the greater the work done by the saliva, the lighter will be the task remaining for the other secretions and the greater the probability of its complete accomplishment."

Oxalic acid diluted to 1 part in 10,000 completely arrests the action of ptyalin. There is sufficient acetic acid in one or two teaspoonfuls of vinegar to entirely suspend salivary digestion. The acids of tomatoes, berries, oranges, grapefruits, lemons, limes, pineapples, sour apples, sour grapes, and other sour fruits are sufficient to destroy the ptyalin of the saliva and suspend starch digestion. Without, apparently understanding why, Dr. Percy Howe of Harvard, says: "Many people who cannot eat oranges at a meal derive great benefit from eating them fifteen to thirty minutes before the meal."

All physiologists agree that acids, even mild acids, destroy ptyalin. Unless and until it can be shown that saliva is capable of digesting starch without the presence of ptyalin, we shall have to continue to insist that acid-starch combinations are indigestible. The blatant assertion by men who never made a serious study of the subject of human nutrition, that any combination of foodstuffs that you like or desire is all right is based on ignorance or prejudice or is just an expression of bigotry.

Our rule, then, should be: *Eat* acids *and starches at separate meals.*

PROTEIN-STARCH COMBINATIONS

Chittenden showed that free hydrochloric acid to the extent of only 0.003 percent is sufficient to suspend the starch-splitting (amylolytic) action of ptyalin, and a slight further increase in acidity not only stops the action, but also destroys the enzyme. In his *Textbook of Physiology* Howell says of *gastric* lipase that, *"this lipase* is *readily destroyed by an* acidity *of 0.2 percent HCl, so that if it* is *of functional importance in gastric digestion its action, like that of ptyalin, must* be *confined to the early* period *of* digestion *before the contents of the stomach have reached their normal* acidity." (Italics mine.) We are not here concerned with the destruction of the *lipase* by the hydrochloric acid of the stomach, but with the destruction of ptyalin by the same acid.

The physiologist Stiles says: "The acid which is highly favorable to gastric digestion, for example, is quite prohibitive to salivary digestion." He says of pepsin, "the power to digest proteins is manifested only with an acid reaction, and is permanently lost when the mixture is made distinctly alkaline. The conditions which permit peptic digestion to take place are, therefore, precisely those which exclude the action of saliva." He declares of the salivary enzyme, ptyalin, "the enzyme is extremely sensitive to acid. Inasmuch as the gastric juice is decidedly acid, it used to be claimed that salivary digestion could not proceed in the stomach." Gastric juice destroys ptytalin and thereby stops starch digestion. This being true, how are we ever to digest our starch foods?

The answer to this question is found in the power of the digestive system to adapt its secretions to the digestive requirements of particular foods, providing, of course, that we respect the limitations of this adaptive mechanism. Dr. Richard C. Cabot of Harvard, who was neither advocating nor combating any special method of food combining, wrote: "When we eat carbohydrates the stomach secretes an *appropriate* juice, a gastric juice of different composition from that which it secretes if it finds proteins coming down. This is a response to the particular demand that is made on the stomach. It is one of the numerous examples of choice or intelligent guidance carried on by parts of the body which are ordinarily thought of as unconscious and having no soul or choice of their own." Here is the secret: *The stomach* secretes a *different kind of* juice *when we eat a starch food from what it secretes when we eat a protein food.*

Pavlov has shown that each kind of food calls forth a particular activity of the digestive glands; that the power of the juice varies with the quality of the food; that special modifications of the activity of the glands are required by different foods; that the strongest juice is poured out when most needed. When bread is eaten little hydrochloric acid is poured into the stomach. The juice secreted upon bread is almost neutral in reaction. When the starch of the bread is digested, much hydrochloric acid is then poured into the stomach to digest the protein of the bread. The two processes - do not go on simultaneously with great efficiency. On the contrary, the secretions are nicely and minutely adjusted, both as to character and to timing, to the varying needs of the complex food substance.

Herein lies the answer to those who object to food combining because "nature combines various food substances in the same food." There is a great difference between the digestion of a *food,* however complex its composition, and the digestion of a *mixture of different foods.* To a single article of food that is a starch protein combination, the body can easily adjust its juices, both as to strength and timing, to the digestive requirements of the food. But when two foods are eaten with different, even opposite digestive needs, this precise adjustment of juices to requirements becomes impossible. If bread and flesh are eaten together, instead of an almost neutral gastric juice being poured into the stomach during the first two hours of digestion, a highly acid juice will be poured out immediately and starch digestion will come to an almost abrupt end.

It should never be lost sight of that physiologically, the first steps in the digestion of starches and proteins take place in opposite media – starch requiring an alkaline medium, protein requiring an acid medium in which to digest. On this point, V.H. Mottram, professor of physiology in the University of London, says in his *Physiology* that, when the food in the stomach comes in contact with the gastric juice, no salivary digestion is possible. He says: "Now gastric juice digests protein and saliva digests starch. Therefore it is obvious that for efficient digestion the meat (protein) part of a meal should come first and the starch part second - just indeed as by instinct is usually the case. Meat precedes pudding as being the most economical procedure."

Mottram explains this matter by saying: "The distal end of the stomach is that in which the churning movement that mixes the food with the gastric juice takes place ... But the food in the quiescent end is still under the influence of the saliva, while the food in the motile end comes in contact with the acid gastric juice and no salivary action is possible." This simply means that if you eat your protein first and your starch last, that the protein will digest in the lower end of the stomach while the starch will digest in its upper end.

If we assume that there is any line of demarcation between the food in the stomach, as his proposition demands, it is still true that, people in general, neither instinctively nor otherwise, consume their proteins and starches in this manner. Perhaps in England it is customary to eat meat at the beginning of a meal and pudding at the end, just as we have a similar practice of taking a dessert at the end of a meal in this country, but it is likely to be the practice there as here, to eat starch and protein together. When the average man or woman eats eggs or cheese, he or she takes bread with the protein. Hot dogs, hamburgers, eggs and toast, beans and rice, and other similar combinations of protein and starch represent the common practice of eating such foods.[2] With such eating, the protein and starch are thoroughly mixed in both ends of the stomach.

Howell makes a somewhat similar statement. He says: "A question of practical importance is as to how far salivary digestion affects the starchy foods under usual circumstances. The chewing process in the mouth thoroughly mixes the food and saliva, or should do so, but the bolus is swallowed much too quickly to enable the enzyme to complete its action. In the stomach the gastric juice is sufficiently acid to destroy the ptyalin, and it was therefore supposed formerly that salivary digestion is promptly arrested on the entrance of food into the stomach, and is normally of but little value as a digestive process. Later knowledge regarding the conditions of the stomach shows on the contrary, that some of the food in an ordinary meal may remain in the fundic end of the stomach for an hour or more untouched by the acid secretion. There is every reason to believe, therefore that salivary digestion may be carried on in the stomach to an important extent."

It is obvious that salivary digestion may be carried on in the stomach to an important extent only in a small part of the food eaten, providing the eating is the usual haphazard mixtures of bread with meat, bread with eggs, bread with cheese, bread with other protein, or potatoes with proteins. When someone eats a sandwich, he does not eat the protein first and then follow with his bun.[3] They are eaten together and thoroughly chewed and mixed together and swallowed together. The stomach has no mechanism for separating these thoroughly intermixed substances and partitioning them off in separate compartments in its cavity.

Mixing foods in this manner is not seen in nature - animals tending to eat but one food at a meal. The carnivore certainly does not mix starches with his proteins. Birds tend to consume insects at one period of the day and seeds at another time. This is certainly the best plan for man to follow, for, at best, the plan suggested by Mottram cannot give ideal results. On the basis of the physiological facts which have been here presented, we offer our second rule for food combining. It is this: *Eat protein foods and carbohydrate foods at* separate *meals*.

By this is meant that cereals, bread, potatoes and other starch foods, should be eaten separately from eggs, cheese, nuts and other protein foods.[4]

PROTEIN-PROTEIN COMBINATIONS

Two proteins of different character and different composition, and associated with other and different food factors call for different modifications of the digestive secretions and different timing of the secretions in order to digest them efficiently. For example, the strongest juice is poured out upon milk in the last hour of digestion, upon flesh in the first hour. Is there no significance in the timing of the secretions thus seen? In our eating practices we habitually ignore such facts and our physiologists have not attached any importance to such matters. Eggs receive the strongest secretion at a different time to that received by either flesh or milk. It is logical, therefore, to assume that eggs should not be taken with milk.[5] It is not too late to recall the harm that was done to tubercular patients by feeding them the abominable combination of eggs and milk. It may be noted in passing that for centuries orthodox Jews have refrained from taking flesh and milk at the same meal.

The fact is that the digestive process is modified to meet the digestive requirements of each protein food and it is impossible for this to be modified in such a manner as to meet the requirements of two different proteins at the same meal. This may not mean that two different kinds of legumes may not be taken together or that two different kinds of nuts may not be taken at the same time; but it certainly means that such protein combinations as beans and eggs, eggs and milk, eggs and nuts, cheese and nuts, milk and nuts, etc., should not be taken.[6] One protein food at a meal will certainly assure greater efficiency in digestion.

Our rule, then, should be: *Eat but* one *concentrated protein food at* a *meal.*

An objection has been offered to this rule that is as follows: the various proteins vary so greatly in their amino-acid content and the body required adequate quantities of certain of these so that, it is necessary to consume more than one protein in order to assure an adequate supply of amino-acids. But inasmuch as most people eat more than one meal a day and there is protein in almost everything we eat, this objection is invalid. One does not have to consume all of his protein at anyone meal.

ACID-PROTEIN COMBINATIONS

The active work of splitting up (digesting) complex protein substances into simpler substances, which takes place in the stomach and which forms the first step in the digestion of proteins, is accomplished by the enzyme, *pepsin.* Pepsin acts only in an acid medium; its action is stopped by alkali. The gastric juice ranges all the way from nearly neutral to strongly acid, depending upon what kind of food is put into the stomach. When proteins are eaten the gastric juice is acid, for it must furnish a favorable medium for the action of *pepsin.*

Because pepsin is active only in an acid medium, the mistake has been made of assuming that the taking of acids with the meal will assist in the digestion of protein. Actually, on the contrary, these acids inhibit the outpouring of gastric juice and thus interfere with the digestion of proteins. Drug acids and fruit acids demoralize gastric digestion, either by destroying the *pepsin,* or by inhibiting its secretion. Gastric juice is not poured out in the presence of acid in the mouth and stomach. The renowned Russian physiologist, Pavlov, positively demonstrated the demoralizing influence of acids upon digestion - both fruit acids and the acid end-results of fermentation. Acid fruits by inhibiting the flow of gastric juice - an unhampered flow of which is imperatively demanded by protein digestion - seriously handicaps protein digestion and results in putrefaction.

The normal stomach secretes all the acid required by *pepsin* in digesting a reasonable quantity of protein. An abnormal stomach may secrete too much acid (hyperacidity) or an insufficient amount (hypoacidity). In either case, taking acids with proteins does not aid digestion. While *pepsin* is not active except in the presence of hydrochloric acid (I can find no evidence that other acids activate this enzyme), excessive gastric acidity prevents its action. Excess acid destroys the *pepsin.*

Based on these simple facts of the physiology of digestion, our rule should be: *Eat proteins and acids at separate meals.*

When we consider the actual process of protein digestion in the stomach and the positive inhibiting effects of acids upon gastric secretion, we realize at once the fallacy of consuming pineapple juice or grapefruit juice or tomato juice with flesh, as advocated by certain so-called dietitians, and the fallacy of beating up eggs in orange juice to make the so-called "pep-cocktail," advocated by other pseudo-dietitians.

Lemon juice, vinegar or other acid used on salads, or added to salad dressing, and eaten with a protein meal, serve as a severe check to hydrochloric secretion and thus interfere with protein digestion.

Although nuts or cheese with acid fruits do not constitute ideal combinations, we may make exceptions to the foregoing rule in the case of these two articles of food. Nuts and cheese containing, as they do considerable oil and fat (cream), are about the only exceptions to the rule that *when acids* are *taken with protein, putrefaction* occurs. These foods do not decompose as quickly as other protein foods when they are not immediately digested. Furthermore, acids do not delay the digestion of nuts and cheese because these foods contain enough fat to inhibit gastric secretion for a longer time than do acids.

FAT -PROTEIN COMBINATIONS

McLeod's *Physiology* in *Modern Medicine* says: "Fat has been shown to exert a distinct inhibiting influence on the secretion of gastric juice ... the presence of oil in the stomach delays the secretion of juice poured out on a subsequent meal of otherwise readily digestible food." Here is an important physiological truth, the full significance of which has seldom been realized. Most men and women who write on food combining ignore the depressing effect fat has upon gastric secretion.

The presence of fat in the food lessens the amount of appetite secretion that is poured into the stomach, lessens the amount of "chemical secretion" poured out, lessens the activity of the gastric glands, lowers the amount of pepsin and hydrochloric acid in the gastric juice and may lower gastric tone by as much as fifty percent. This inhibiting effect may last two or more hours.

This means that when protein food is eaten, fat should not be taken at the same meal. In other words, such foods as cream, butter, oils of various kinds, gravies, etc., should not be consumed at the same meal with nuts, cheese, eggs, legumes.[7] It will be noted, in this connection, that those foods that normally contain fat within themselves, as nuts or cheese or milk, require longer time to digest than those protein foods that are lacking in fat.

Our fourth rule, then, is: *Eat fats and proteins at separate meals.*

It is well to know that an abundance of green vegetables, especially un-cooked ones, counteract the inhibiting effect of fat, so that if one must have fat with one's protein, one may offset its inhibiting effect upon the digestion of protein by consuming much green substance with the meal.

SUGAR-PROTEIN COMBINATION

All sugars - commercial sugars, syrups, sweet fruits, honey, etc., - have an inhibiting effect upon the secretion of gastric juice and upon the motility of the stomach. This fact adds significance to the remark made to children by mothers that the eating of cookies before meals "spoils the appetite." Sugars taken with protein hinder protein digestion.

Sugars undergo no digestion in the mouth and stomach. They are digested in the intestine. If taken alone they are not held in the stomach long, but are quickly sent into the intestine. When eaten with other foods, either proteins or starches, they are held up in the stomach for a prolonged period, awaiting the digestion of the other foods. While thus awaiting the completion of protein or starch digestion they undergo fermentation.

Based on these simple facts of digestion, our rule is: *Eat sugars and pro-teins at separate meals.*

SUGAR-STARCH COMBINATIONS

Starch digestion normally begins in the mouth and continues, under proper conditions, for some time in the stomach. Sugars do not undergo any digestion in either the mouth or stomach, but in the small intestine only. When consumed alone sugars are quickly sent out of the stomach into the intestine. When consumed with other foods, they are held up in the stomach for some time awaiting the digestion of the other foods. As they tend to ferment very quickly under the conditions of warmth and moisture existing in the stomach, this type of eating almost guarantees acid fermentation.

Jellies, jams, fruit butters, commercial sugar (white or brown, beet, cane or lactic), honey, molasses, syrups, etc., added to cakes, breads, pastries, cereals, potatoes, etc., *produce* fermentation. The regularity with which millions of our people eat cereals and sugar for breakfast and suffer with sour stomach, sour eructations, and other evidences of indigestion as a consequence, would be amusing were it not so tragic. Sweet fruits with starch also result in fermentation. Breads containing dates, raisins, figs, etc., so popular among the frequenters of the "health food" store, are dietetic abominations. In many quarters it is thought that if honey is used instead of sugar this may be avoided, but such is not the case. Honey with hot cakes, syrup with hot cakes, etc., are almost sure to ferment.

There is every reason to believe that the presence of the sugar with the starch definitely interferes with the digestion of starch. When sugar is taken into the mouth there is a copious outpouring of saliva, but it contains no ptyalin for ptyalin does not act upon sugar. If the starch is disguised with sugar, honey, syrup, jellies, jams, etc., this will prevent the adaptation of the saliva to starch digestion. Little or no ptyalin will be secreted and starch digestion will not take place.

Major Reginald F. E. Austin, M.B., RAM.C., M.R.C.S., L.R.C.P., says: "foods that are wholesome by themselves or in certain combinations often disagree when eaten with others. For example, bread and butter taken together cause no unpleasantness, but if sugar or jam or marmalade is added, trouble may follow. Because the sugar will be taken up first, and the conversion of the starch into sugar is then delayed. Mixtures of starch and sugar invite fermentation and its attendant evils."

Upon these facts we base the rule: *Eat starches and sugars at separate meals.*

EATING MELONS

Large numbers of people complain that melons do not agree with them. Some of these people, desiring to appear more up-to-date in their knowledge, explain that they are *allergic* to melons. I have fed melons in quantity to hundreds of such people and found that they have no trouble with them and that their supposed *allergy* was but a figment of the imagination. Melons are such wholesome foods and are so easy of digestion that even the most feeble digestions can handle them very nicely.

But trouble, frequently severe suffering, does often follow the eating of melons. Why? These foods undergo no digestion in the stomach. The little digestion they require takes place in the intestine. If taken properly, they are retained in the stomach but a few minutes and are then passed into the intestine. But if taken with other foods that require a lengthy stay in the stomach for salivary or gastric digestion, they are held up in the stomach. As they decompose very quickly when cut open and kept in a warm place, they are prone to give rise to much gas and discomfort when eaten with most other foods.

I take a person who says that every time he eats watermelon he has severe pain in his abdomen, that he fills up with gas, and that he suffers in other ways. He declares that melons have always "disagreed" with him, that he could never eat them. I feed this person an abundance of melon and he has no gas, no pain, no discomfort. How do I achieve this? I feed the melon alone. He is given all the melon he desires at a meal - makes his meal on melon. He immediately discovers that melons do "agree" with him, that he is not allergic to melons.

From these facts we derive the rule: *Eat melons alone.*

This means that watermelons, honey dews, musk melons, cantaloupes, casabas, persian melons, banana melons, Crenshaw melons, pie melons, Christmas melons, and other melons should be eaten alone. They should not be eaten between meals, but at meal time. It is well to make the meal on melon. I have tried feeding melons with fresh fruits and there seems to be no reason why they may not be fed together, if this is desired.

TAKE MILK ALONE

It is the rule in nature that the young of each species takes its milk alone. Indeed, in the early life of young mammals, they take no other food but milk. Then there comes a time when they eat milk and other foods, but they takecthem separately. Finally, there comes a time when they are weaned, after which, they never take milk again. Milk is the food of the young. There is no need for it after the end of the normal suckling period. The dairy industry and the medical profession have taught us that we need a quart of milk a day so long as we live - we are never to be weaned but are to remain sucklings all our lives. This is a commercial program and expresses no human need.

Due to its protein and fat (cream) content, milk combines poorly with all foods. It will combine fairly well with acid fruits. The first thing that occurs when it enters the stomach is that it coagulates - forms curds. These curds tend to form around the particles of other food in the stomach thus insulating them against the gastric juice. This prevents their digestion until after the milk curd is digested.

Our rule with milk is: *Take milk alone* or *let it alone.*

In feeding milk to young children a fruit meal may be fed and then, half an hour afterward, milk may be given. The milk should not be given with the fruits, except in the case of acid fruits. The orthodox Jew follows a very excellent plan of eating when he refuses to consume milk with flesh. But its use with cereals orother starch is equally as objectionab

DESSERTS

Desserts eaten at the end of a meal, usually after the eater has eaten to repletion, very commonly after he has eaten more than he requires of other foods, are such things as cakes, pies, puddings, ice cream, stewed fruits, etc., which combine badly with almost every other part of the meal. They serve no useful purpose and are not advisable. There should be but one rule with reference to them; it is this: *Desert the desserts.*

Dr. Tilden used to advise that if you must have a piece of pie, eat the pie and a large raw vegetable salad and nothing else, and then miss *the next* meal. Dr. Harvey W. Wiley once remarked that the food value of pie is unquestioned; "it only remains to be digested." Certainly, eaten with a regular meal, as is the custom, it is not well digested. The same may be said for the other desserts. Cold desserts, like ice cream, interpose another barrier to the digestive process - that of cold.

NORMAL DIGESTION

I n his *Textbook of Physiology* Howell says that "In the large intestine protein putrefaction is a constant and normal occurrence." He records that "Recognizing that fermentation by means of bacteria is a normal occurrence in the gastro-intestinal canal, the question has arisen whether this process is in any way necessary to normal digestion and nutrition." After considerable discussion of this question and reference to experiments that have been made he reaches no definite conclusion, but thinks "it seems wise to take the conservative *view* that while the presence of the bacteria confers no positive benefit, the organism has adapted itself under usual conditions to neutralize their injurious action."

He points out that the putrefactive bacteria break down the proteins into amino-acids, but that they do not stop here. They destroy the amino-acids, and give us, as final products of their activities, such poisons as indol, skatol, phenol, phenylpropionic and phenylacetic acids, fatty acids, carbon dioxide, hydrogen, marsh gas, hydrogen sulphide, etc. He adds that "many of these products are given off in the feces, while others are absorbed in part and excreted subsequently in the urine." Finally, he says: "There is evidence that other more or less toxic substances belonging to the group of amines are produced by the further action of the bacteria on the amino-acids in the protein molecule."

It does not seem logical to assume that such a process of toxin formation is either normal or necessary in the process of digestion. It seems to me that Howell and the other physiologists have merely mistaken a common or almost universal occurrence, at least it is almost universal in civilized life, as a normal occurrence. They have not stopped to ask why fermentation and putrefaction occur in the digestive tract. What causes it to occur? That it is a source of poisoning they admit. Howell goes so far as to say: "It is well known that excessive bacterial action may lead to intestinal troubles, such as diarrhea, or possibly to more serious interference with general nutrition owing to the formation of toxic products, such as the amines." He fails to define what he means by "excessive bacterial action."

I have repeatedly pointed out the folly of accepting mere conventions as normal. The mere fact that protein putrefaction is well nigh universal in the colons of civilized man is, by itself, not sufficient to establish the phenomenon as a normal one. It is first necessary to ask and answer the question: *Why* is *protein putrefaction* so common? It may also be well to ask if it serves any useful purpose.

Are the putrefaction and fermentation that are so common due to overeating, to the eating of illegitimate proteins, to eating wrong combinations, to eating under physical and emotional conditions (fatigue, work, worry, fear, anxiety, pain, fever, inflammation, etc.) that retard or suspend digestion? Is it the result of impaired digestion from any cause? Must we always take it for granted that the present eating practice of civilized man are normal? Why must we accept as normal what we find in a race of sick and weakened beings?

Foul stools, loose stools, impacted stools, pebbly stools, much foul gas, colitis, hemorrhoids, bleeding with stools, the need for toilet paper, and all the other things of this nature that accompany present-day living, are swept into the orbit of the normal by the assertion that putrefaction is a normal occurrence in the human colon. We have it asserted in different words that "whatever is, is right."

That there are animals that do not present protein putrefaction in their intestinal tracts, that there are men and women whose eating and living habits give odorless stools and no gas, that a change of habits produces a change of results - these facts are of no importance to physiologists who are devoted to the stultifying axiom that only conventions are to be received as data. Howell accepts as normal the generally prevailing septic condition of the human colon and completely ignores the causes that produce and maintain this condition of sepsis.

The blood stream should receive from the digestive tract water, amino-acids, fatty acids, glycerol, monosaccharides, minerals and vitamins. It should not receive alcohol, acetic acid ptomaines, leucomaines, hydrogen sulphide, etc. Nutritive materials not poisons, should be received from the digestive tract.

When starches and complex sugars are digested they are broken down into simple sugars called monosaccharides, which are usable substances - *nutriments*. When starches and sugars undergo fermentation they are broken down into carbon dioxide, acetic acid, alcohol and water, which substances, with the exception of water, are non-usable substances - poisons. When proteins are digested, they are broken down into amino-acids, which are usable substances - *nutrients*. When proteins putrefy, they are broken down into a variety of ptomaines and leucomaines, which are non-usable substances - poisons. So with all other food factors, enzymic digestion of foods prepares them for use by the body; bacterial decomposition of foods unfits them for use by the body. The first process gives us nutrient elements as the finished product; the second process *gives* us poisons as the end-result.

What avails it to consume the theoretically required number of calories daily, only to *have* the food ferment and putrefy in the digestive tract? Food that thus spoils does not yield up its calories to the body. What is gained by eating abundantly of adequate proteins only to have these putrefy in the gastro-intestinal canal? Proteins thus rendered unfit for entrance into the body do not yield up their amino-acids. What benefit does one receive from eating vitamin-rich foods only to have these decompose in the stomach and intestines? Foods thus rotted do not supply the body with vitamins. What nutritive good comes from eating mineral-laden foods only to have these rot in the alvine canal? Foods that are thus rendered unfit for use provide the body with no minerals. Carbohydrates that ferment in the digestive tract are converted into alcohol and acetic acid, not into monosaccharides. Fats that become rancid in the stomach and intestine provide the body with no fatty acids and glycerol. To derive sustenance from the foods eaten, they must be digested; they must not rot.

Discussing phenol, indol and skatol, Howell points out that phenol (carbolic acid), after it is absorbed, is combined in part, with sulphuric acid, forming an etheral sulphate, or phenolsulphonic acid, and is excreted in the urine in this form. "So also with cresol," he adds. Indol and skatol, after being absorbed, are oxidized into indoxyl and skatoxyl, after which they are combined with sulphuric acid, like phenol, and are excreted in the urine as indoxyl-sulphuric acid and skatoxyl-sulphuric acid. These poisons have long been found in the urine and the amount of them occuring in the urine is taken as an index to the extent of putrefaction that is going on in the intestine. That the body may and does establish toleration for these poisons, as it does for other poisons that are habitually introduced into it is certain, but it seems the height of folly to assume that "the organism has adapted itself under usual conditions to neutralize" these products of bacterial activity. Certainly the discomfort that arises from the accumulation of gas in the abdomen, the bad breath that grows out of gastro-intestinal fermentation and putrefaction, the foul and unpleasant odor from the stools and from the expelled gasses are as undesirable as are the poisons.

That it is possible to have a clean sweet breath, freedom from gas pressure and odorless stools is common knowledge. It seems to me that instead of assuming that a common phenomenon is normal, perhaps even necessary, it were wise to consider the causes of this occurrence and determine whether or not it is normal. If it is possible to avoid the unpleasant results of fermentation and putrefaction, if it is possible to avoid the poisoning that results from these, if we can remove from the body the burden of oxidizing and eliminating these bacterial products, it seems to me to be eminently desirable to do so. If it is admitted that "excessive bacterial activity" may produce diarrhea and even serious nutritional evils, what may we expect from long continued bacterial activity that is short of "excessive"? This, it seems to me, is a pertinent question.

Anything that reduces digestive power, anything that slows up the processes of digestion, anything that temporarily suspends the digestive process will favor bacterial activity. Such things as over eating (eating beyond enzymic capacity), eating when fatigued, eating just before beginning work, eating when chilled or over heated, eating when feverish, in pain, when there is severe inflammation, when not hungry, when worried, anxious, fearful, angry, etc. - eating under all of these and similar circumstances favors bacterial decomposition of the foods eaten. The use of condiments, vinegar, alcohol, and other substances that retard digestion favors bacterial decomposition of the foods eaten. The use of condiments, vinegar, alcohol and other substances that retard digestion favors bacterial activity. If we carefully analyze the eating practices of most civilized people, we may easily find a hundred and one reasons why gastro-intestinal fermentation and putrefaction are so nearly universal without assuming that these processes are normal, perhaps necessary. The causes of digestive inefficiency and failure are legion.

One of the most common causes of digestive inefficiency, one that is almost universally practiced in this country, is eating wrong combinations of foods. The almost universal practice of ignoring our enzymic limitations and eating haphazardly is responsible for a large part of the indigestion with which almost everybody suffers more or less constantly. The proof of this lies in the fact that feeding correct combinations ends the indigestion. This statement should not be misunderstood. Feeding correct combinations will only improve and not end indigestion, if the indigestion is due in part to other causes. If worry, for example, is a prominent factor in cause, worry will have to be discontinued before digestion can be normal. But it should be known that worry with wrong combinations will give worse indigestion that worry with correct combinations.

Rex Beach, who once mined gold in Alaska, wrote of gold miners: "We ate greatly of baking-powder bread, underdone beans and fat pork. No sooner were these victuals down than they went to war on us. The real call of the wild was not the howl of the timber wolf, the maniac laughter of the Arctic loon, or the mating cry of the bull moose; it was the dyspeptic belch of the miner." Our physiologists, ignoring the mode of eating that is responsible for it, would declare this "belch of the miner," his abdominal distension and distress, the resulting gastro-intestinal decomposition, foul stools and passing of much foul gas, to be normal. If the miner did not have Bell-ans or Alka-Seltzer with which to palliate his distress and encourage further indiscretions in eating, he could always run his finger down his throat and induce vomiting, if his distress became too great. Constipation, alternating with diarrhea, was common on such a diet.

Millions of dollars are spent yearly for drugs which afford a temporary respite from the discomfort and distress that result from decomposition of food in the stomach and intestine. Substances to neutralize acidity, to absorb gas, to relieve pain, even to relieve headache due to gastric irritation, are employed by train loads by the American people. Other substances, such as pepsin, are employed to aid in the digestion of food. Instead of regarding this as a normal condition, *Hygienists* regard it as an extremely abnormal condition. Ease and comfort, not pain and distress, are marks of health. Normal digestion is not accompanied with any signs or symptoms of disease.

How to Take
Your Proteins

A nd Jehovah spake unto Moses, saying "I have heard the murmurs of the children of Israel: speak unto them, saying' At evening ye shall eat flesh, and in the morning ye shall be filled with bread.'" "And Moses said ... 'Jehovah shall give you in the evening, flesh to eat, and in the morning, bread to the full.' " Thus did the murmurings of the children of Israel in the wilderness cause to be set down in the ancient book a record of an eating practice, which although' lost to us with the passage of time, has been revived today on physiological grounds - that of eating protein and carbohydrate foods at separate meals. It is interesting in this connection, also to note that Tilden gave it as his opinion that there should be twelve hours between the eating of a protein and a starch meal. The foregoing account says nothing about what was eaten with the flesh, but in the instructions for the eating of the feast of the Passover, it will be noted that an abundance of green herbs was prescribed along with the lamb flesh. Green vegetables combine best with protein foods. We have learned that it is best to eat proteins and carbohydrates at separate meals. The processes of digestion of these two types of foods are so different that they do not take place with any degree of efficiency in the same digestive cavity at the same time. This is so contrary to popular practice that it will require considerable explanation.

Digestion is a physiological process in which the body varies its activities according to many factors and in keeping with the character of the viands that it is engaged in reducing to suitable materials. A remarkable fact is noted concerning the work of the digestive glands: namely, the digestive tract can vary its fluids and enzymes to suit these to the character of the food eaten. The following words are quoted from the second edition (1961) of a *Textbook of Medical Physiology* by Arthur C. Guyton, a standard text: " ... .in some portions of the gastrointestinal tract even the types of enzymes or other constituents of the secretions are varied in relation to the type of the food present."

Perhaps Pavlov laid greatest stress upon this ability of the digestive tube to vary its fluids and enzymes in keeping with the types of food eaten, although some knowledge of the fact existed prior to his investigations. The fact is generally known to physiologists today, although neither Pavlov nor any other physiologist has ever attempted to make any practical application of it to everyday life. Indeed, physiology seems to be looked upon as a "pure science," not as one that has any practical bearing on the everyday life of man.

The variations in the enzymic and other constituents of the digestive secretions in the presence of different foods is an effort to make the digestive juices conform to the requirements of digestion of the different foods. These variations include variations in the alkalinity and acidity (pH) of the secretions, variations in the concentration of the enzymes, timing of the secretions, etc., in fitting them to the different foods.

The suiting of the juices and their enzymic content to the character of the food eaten is possible, however, only when the foods eaten are not so radically different that the juices required or the timing of their secretion conflicts with one another. These variations in the acid-alkaline character of the secretion, the enzymic concentration and in the timing of the secretions can have meaning only if the food is eaten alone or is eaten with other foods that do not conflict with the digestive processes required to digest a particular food.

This ability of the digestive tube to vary its secretions to meet the digestive requirements of a food explains how it can efficiently handle a food, such as a potato, a grain or a legume, which is a starch-protein combination, providing the potato or grain or legume is eaten alone or with foods that do not make the adaptation of the juice to the food impossible. Potatoes with flesh or with cheese, or flesh with bread, both being protein-carbohydrate combinations, are not, however, handled with the same efficiency for the reason that the juices cannot be adapted to the needs of two foods of such opposite character.

It is one thing to eat one food, however complex its nature; it is quite another thing to eat two foods of "opposite" character. The digestive juices can be readily adapted to one food, such as cereals, that is a protein-starch combination, but they cannot be well adapted to two foods, such as bread and cheese. How true it is, as Dr. Tilden used to say, that nature never produced a sandwich. It should be obvious that the human digestive tract is adapted to the digestion of natural food combinations, but it is certainly not adapted to the digestion of the haphazard and indiscriminate mixtures that are eaten by the civilized person of today. Natural combinations offer but little difficulty to the digestive system. Deadly perils arise out of mixtures of incompatibles, such as a Thanksgiving or Christmas dinner, or the chicken pie, cocktails (even with spirits omitted), punch, pastry, bread and other substances eaten at a church festival. Such a bacchanalian feast often ends in an epidemic of "ptomaine poisoning," in diptheria, measles, etc.

An indiscriminate and haphazard mixture of foods, such as is commonly eaten by the average person, at his or her regular mealtime, precludes the possibility that any possible variation in the character of the digestive secretions poured out upon the meal will render the digestion of the meal efficient. It is for this reason that we advise such food combinations as offer least conflict in the process of digestion - that we respect our enzymic limitations.

In their *Principles of Biochemistry* (1959), a standard text, White, Handler, Smith and Stetten say: "The part played by saliva in digestion of starch in the intact mammal is uncertain owing to the variable durations of contact of enzyme and substrate. The mixing of the bolus of food with the acid gastric juice undoubtedly interrupts the action of the salivary amylase, since this enzyme is inactivated at low pH values. Only in individuals deficient in secretion of gastric Hcl may salivary digestion be presumed to continue in the stomach."

The fact here portrayed: namely, that the hydrochloric acid of the gastric juice inactivates or actually destroys salivary amylase or ptyalin in the stomach is well known to physiologists and physiological chemists, but they commonly gloss over it instead of frankly recognizing, as do the foregoing authors, that salivary digestion soon ends when food reaches the stomach. Arthur K. Anderson, in his *Essentials of Physiological Chemistry* (1961), after duly recognizing this fact, seeks to escape from its plain implications by saying that "since salivary amylase acts until the pH reaches 4.0, it is evident that considerable action may take place in the stomach before acidity develops sufficiently to inhibit it, . . .It has been estimated that amylase activity may continue for thirty minutes after food is swallowed ..."

Repetitions of Anderson's tests made in the laboratory, using a standard pH meter, showed absolutely no amylase activity at a pH of 4 and only the slightest activity at a pH of 5. From this fact I would say that amylase activity is inhibited in the stomach earlier than Anderson thinks. Tests have shown that hydrochloric acid added to the food arrests the action of the ptyalin in sixty seconds. The acidity of the stomach juice is a factor to be considered, not merely as the acid juice gradually penetrates the food bolus, but from the swallowing of the first bite of food.

In the 1961 edition of the *Physiological Basis of Medical Practice,* the physiologists, Best and Taylor, say: "The salivary amylase requires for its activity an alkaline, neutral or faintly acid medium; therefore, it was thought that the higher acid gastric juice would prevent, or soon terminate salivary digestion. It has been shown, however, that the latter part of the meal, which usually consists of carbohydrates, may remain in the fundus of the stomach, protected for some time from the action of the gastric juice, by a layer of food ingested previously

. . .For this reason it is likely that under favorable circumstances considerable digestion of starch is accomplished during this period ..."

The unconscious self-deception of these physiologists is evident at first sight. The carbohydrate that is more or less regularly eaten at the end of a meal is the dessert and this is commonly a sugar which requires no salivary digestion. People do not, as a common practice, eat their proteins at the beginning of the meal and their starches at the end. They eat them together, as in the familiar eating of bread and flesh together in a hamburger. Flesh and bread, bread and eggs, flesh and potatoes or flesh and peas are common mixtures.

If the physiologist is satisfied with "considerable starch digestion" in the upper end of the stomach, while the starch in the rest of the stomach is not digested, I presume that he may be satisfied with the deficient digestion that occurs when the common mixtures are eaten, but for the man or woman who wants efficient digestion, such mixtures should not be considered. The statement made by Anderson that "any starch which has not been hydrolyzed in the mouth and stomach by salivary amylase is digested in the intestine by pancreatic amylase," is contradicted by the great amount of undigested starch that is found in the stools of those who mix their proteins and carbohydrates.

Highly acid gastric juices are secreted with which to digest protein foods, but if starch is taken without protein the gastric juice may be either alkaline, neutral or weakly acid. Even if the starch contains protein, as it does if potatoes, grains or legumes are eaten, the acid secretion is timed so that it is poured out upon the food after salivary digestion of starch is completed. If we would but keep our protein meals and our starch meals separate, after the ancient pattern, we would enjoy better digestion, hence better health.

As all physiologists are agreed that the character of the digestive juice secreted corresponds with the character of the food to be digested and that each food calls for its own specific modification of the digestive juice, it follows as the night the day, that complex mixtures of foods greatly impair the efficiency of digestion. Simple meals will prove to be more easily digested, hence more healthful.

Conventional eating habits violate all of the rules of food combining that have been given in the preceding chapters and, since the majority of people manage to live for at least a few years and to "enjoy" their aches and pains and their frequent "spells of sickness," few of them are willing to give any intelligent consideration to their eating habits. They usually declare, when the subject of food combining comes up, that they eat all of the condemned combinations regularly and it does not hurt them. Life and death, health and disease are mere matters of accident to them. Unfortunately they are encouraged in this view by their medical advisers.

More than sixty years spent in feeding the well and the sick, the weak and the strong, the old and the young, have demonstrated that a change to correctly combined meals is followed by an immediate improvement in health as a consequence of lightening the load the digestive organs have to carry, thus assuring better digestion, improved nutrition and less poisoning. I know that such meals are followed by less fermentation and less putrefaction, less gas and discomfort. I do not believe that such experiences are worth much if they cannot be explained by correct principles, but I have explained them in preceding pages, so that they do assume great importance. The rules of food combining herein given are soundly rooted in physiology, thoroughly tested by experience, and are worthy of more than a passing thought.

A great part of the yearly massacre of children's tonsils grows out of the constant fermentation in their digestive tracts consequent upon their regular eating a flesh-and-bread, cereals-and-sugar, cookies-and-fruit, etc., diet. Until parents learn how to feed their children with proper respect for enzymic limitations and cease feeding them the so-called "balanced meals" now in vogue, their children are going to continue to suffer, not only with colds and tonsillar troubles, but with gastritis (indigestion), diarrhea, constipation, feverishness, the various *children's* diseases, poliomyelitis, etc.

Commonly eaten combinations are bread and flesh - hot dogs, sandwiches, hamburgers, ham on rye, and the like - bread and eggs, bread and cheese, potatoes and flesh, potatoes and eggs (eggs in potato salad, for example), cereals with eggs (usually at breakfast), etc. Nor is it customary to eat the protein first and the carbohydrate afterwards. These foods are eaten together and thrown into the stomach in the most haphazard and indiscriminate manner. The customary way of eating breakfast is to have cereal first (usually with milk or cream and sugar), and then egg on toast. Viewing the common breakfast, which follows a common pattern eaten by most Americans, we should not be surprised that it is so regularly followed by indigestion, nor that the traffic in Bromo-Seltzer, Alka-Seltzer, Bellans, Tums, baking soda, etc., is carried out on such a large scale.

Dishes of Italian origin that are growing very popular in this country are such mixtures as spaghetti and meat balls, spaghetti and cheese, spaghetti and ravioli. The spaghetti is commonly served with tomato sauce and white bread. A small chopped salad that accompanies, contains olive oil, vinegar and great quantities of salt. Other dressings are often served with the salad. White bread is usually served with this abominable mixture. In the smaller places oleomargarine is served. Beer or wine frequently is taken with such a meal.

The radio hawker tells the poor victims of such unphysiological habits of eating that when he suffers with "acid indigestion," he should resort to some one or other of the popular palliatives - nobody ever hints that such palliation guarantees the continuance of the evil habits and assures the later development of serious trouble. "Great oaks from little acorns grow," runs the old copybook maxim, but in pathology this principle is not recognized by those who presume to know.

Inasmuch as, physiologically, the first step in the digestion of starch and the first step in the digestion of protein takes place in opposite media – starch requiring an alkaline medium, protein requiring an acid medium - these two types of foods certainly should not be eaten at the same meal.

It is well known to physiologists that undigested starch absorbs pepsin. This being true it is inevitable that the eating of starches and proteins at the same meal will retard protein digestion. Tests have shown, it is claimed, that this retardation is not great - protein digestion being retarded but four to six minutes, which is insignificant. There is reason to believe that these findings are faulty. For, if the only results of such a combination is a four to six minutes retardation of the digestion of protein, so much undigested protein should not be found in the stools of those who eat such mixtures. I am convinced that the interference with protein digestion is greater than the tests indicate. Those who object to efforts to properly combine our foods tend to focus attention on the protein and, using the results of these tests as the basis of their objection to the rule against mixing proteins and carbohydrates, they studiously avoid all reference to the suspension of starch digestion that results from such mixtures.

Previously we learned that it is unwise to consume more than one kind of protein at a meal. This is true, not merely because it complicates and retards the digestive process, but also, because it leads to over eating of protein. At present the trend is to over-emphasize the need for protein foods and to encourage overeating of these foods. I would like to enter a warning against this folly at this place and point out that it is a return to the dietary fallacies of half a century ago. Diet fads, indeed, seem to run in circles.

So different in character are the specific secretions poured out upon each different food that Pavlov speaks of "milk juice," "bread juice" and "meat juice." Two proteins of different character and different composition require different types of digestive juices and these juices, of different strength and character are poured into the stomach at different times during the digestive process. Khizhin, one of Pavlov's co-workers, showed that the secretion response of the digestive glands is not "limited to the powers of the juice but extends to the rate of its flow, and also its total quantity." The character of the food eaten determines not only the digestive power of the juice secreted upon it, but also its total acidity - acidity is greatest with flesh, least with bread. There is also a marvelous adjustment of the juice as to timing, the strongest juice being poured out in the first hour with flesh, in the third hour with bread, in the last hour of digestion with milk.

Due to the fact that each separate kind of food determines a definite hourly rate of secretion and occasions characteristic limitations in the various powers of the juices, foods requiring marked differences in the digestive secretions, as, for example, bread and flesh, certainly should not be consumed at the same meal. Pavlov showed that five times as much pepsin is poured out upon bread as upon milk containing an amount of protein equivalent to that contained in the bread, while the nitrogen of flesh requires more pepsin than milk. These different kinds of foods received quantities of enzyme corresponding to the differences in their digestibility. Comparing equivalent weights, flesh requires the most and milk the least amount of gastric juice, but comparing equivalents of nitrogen, bread needs the most and flesh the least juice.

All of these facts are very well known to physiologists, but they have never attempted to make any practical application of them. Indeed, when they condescend to discuss them at all in relation to the practical problems of life (of eating), they tend to gloss over them and to provide flimsy reasons why the haphazard eating practices that are almost everywhere in vogue should be continued. They are inclined to regard the more immediate evil results of such imprudent eating as normal, as was shown in the previous chapter.

Due to the inhibiting effects of acids, sugars and fats upon digestive secretion, it is unwise to eat such foods with proteins. Suppose we consider these combinations briefly in the order given.

The inhibiting effect of fat (butter, cream, oils, oleomargarine, etc.) upon gastric secretion, which retards protein digestion for two hours or more, renders it inadvisable to consume fats with proteins., The presence of fat in fat meats, in fried meats and fried eggs, in milk, nuts and similar foods is the probable reason that these foods require longer to digest than do lean roasts or coddled or poached eggs. Fat meats and fried meats are particularly likely to give the eater trouble. We should make it a rule, therefore, not to eat fats of any kind with our proteins.

The inhibiting effect of fat upon gastric secretion may be counteracted by consuming a plentiful supply of green vegetables, particularly uncooked. Uncooked cabbage is particularly effective in this respect. For this reason, it were better to consume green vegetables with cheese and nuts than to consume acid fruits with them, even though, this latter is not particularly objectionable.

Sugars, by inhibiting both gastric secretion and gastric motility (movement of the stomach) interfere with the digestion of proteins. At the same time these food substances, which require no digestion in the mouth and stomach, are held up pending the digestion of the proteins, hence they undergo fermentation. Proteins should not be eaten at the same meal with sugars of any kind or character. Dr. Phillip Norman's experiments showed that taking cream and sugar after a meal delays the digestion of the meal altogether for several hours.

Acids of all kinds inhibit the secretion of gastric juice. They thus interfere with the digestion of proteins. The exceptions are cheese, nuts and avocados. These foods, containing, as they do, cream and oil which inhibit the secretion of gastric juices as much and as long as do acids, do not have their digestion appreciably interfered with when acids are taken with them.

The foods that combine best with protein foods of all kinds are the non-starchy and succulent vegetables. Spinach, chard, kale, beet greens, mustard greens, turnip greens, Chinese cabbage, broccoli, cabbage, asparagus, fresh green beans, okra, Brussel sprouts, all fresh tender squash, except Hubbard squash, onions, celery, lettuce, cucumbers, radishes, sorrel, water cress, parsley, endive, dandelion, collards, rape, escarole, cardoon, broccoli-de-rappe, bamboo sprouts and similar non-starchy foods.

The following vegetables form poor foods to combine with proteins; beets, turnips, pumpkins, carrots, salsify (vegetable oyster or oyster plant), cauliflower, kohlrabi, rutabagas, beans, peas, Jerusalem artichokes, potatoes, including the sweet potato. These foods being somewhat starchy, they make better additions to the starch meal. Beans and peas, being protein-starch combinations in themselves, are better eaten as a starch or as a protein, combined with green vegetables, without other protein or starch with the meal. Potatoes are sufficiently starchy to form the starch part of the starch meal.

The following menus constitute properly combined protein meals. It is suggested that the protein meal be eaten in the evening. Acids and oils and oily dressing should not be taken with the protein meals. These meals may be eaten in amounts required by the individual.

Vegetable Salad	Vegetable Salad
Green Squash	Chard
Spinach	Asparagus
Nuts	Nuts

Vegetable Salad
Asparagus
Yellow Squash
Nuts

Vegetable Salad
Broccoli
Fresh Corn
Nuts

Vegetable Salad
Okra
Spinach
Nuts

Vegetable Salad
Chard
Yellow Squash
Nuts

Vegetable Salad
Collards
Yellow Squash
Avocado

Vegetable Salad
Mustard Greens
Green Beans
Avocado

Vegetable Salad
Turnip Greens
Green Peas
Avocado

Vegetable Salad
Yellow Squash
Cabbage
Sunflower Seed

Vegetable Salad
Spinach
Broccoli
Sunflower Seed

Vegetable Salad
Chard
Okra
Cottage Cheese

Vegetable Salad
Spinach
Green Squash
Cottage Cheese

Vegetable Salad
Beet Green
Green Peas
Cottage Cheese

Vegetable Salad
Beet Greens
Broccoli
Cottage Cheese

Vegetable Salad
Spinach
Cabbage
Unprocessed Cheese

Vegetable Salad
Baked Eggplant
Chard
Eggs

Vegetable Salad
Spinach
Yellow Squash
Eggs

Vegetable Salad
Beet Greens
String Beans
Nuts[8]

Vegetable Salad
Green Squash
Kale
Unprocessed Cheese

Vegetable Salad
Beet Greens
Okra
Sunflower Seed

Vegetable Salad
Kale
String Beans
Sunflower Seed

Vegetable Salad
Baked Eggplant
Chard
Soy Sprouts

Vegetable Salad
Asparagus
Green Beans
Walnuts

Vegetable Salad
Okra
Beet Greens
Sunflower Seed

Vegetable Salad
Okra
Yellow Squash
Cottage Cheese

Vegetable Salad
Chard
Yellow Squash
Avocado

Vegetable Salad
White Cabbage
Spinach
Nuts

Vegetable Salad
Broccoli
Green Beans
Nuts

Vegetable Salad
Steamed Onions
Swiss Chard
Unprocessed Cheese

Vegetable Salad
Green Squash
Turnip Greens
Soy Sprouts[9]

Vegetable Salad
Red Cabbage
Spinach
Cottage Cheese

Vegetable Salad
Turnip Greens
String Beans
Eggs

Vegetable Salad
Asparagus
Cone Artichokes
Avocado

Vegetable Salad
Baked Eggplant
Kale
Avocado

Vegetable Salad
Okra
Red Cabbage
Avocado

Vegetable Salad
Yellow Squash
Chard
Avocado

Vegetable Salad
Yellow Squash
Mustard Greens
Pecans[10]

HOW TO TAKE
YOUR STARCH

CHAPTER VI

One author says: "Don't serve more than two foods rich in sugar or starch at the same meal. When you serve bread and potatoes, your starch-license has run out. A meal that includes peas, bread, potatoes, sugar, cake and after dinner mints should also include a Vitamin B Complex capsule, some bicarbonate of soda (other than that used on the vegetables), and the address of the nearest specialist in arthritis and other degenerative diseases."

For more than seventy years it has been the rule in *Hygienic* circles to take but one starch at a meal and to consume no sweet foods with the starch meal. Sugars, syrups, honeys, cakes, pies, mints, etc., have been tabu with starches. We do not say to those who come to us for advice: If you eat these with your starches, take a dose of baking soda with them. We tell them to avoid the fermentation that is almost inevitable. In *Hygienic* circles it is considered the height of folly to take a poison and then take an antidote with it. We think it best not to take the poison.

Sugar with starch means fermentation. It means a sour stomach. It means discomfort. Those who are addicted to the honey-eating practice and who are laboring under the popular fallacy that honey is a "natural sweet" and may be eaten indiscriminately, should know that this rule not to take sweets with starches applies to honey as well. Honey or syrup, it makes no difference which, with your cereals, honey or sugar to sweeten your cakes – these combinations spell fermentation. White sugar, brown sugar, "raw" sugar, imitation brown sugar (that is, white sugar that has been colored), black strap molasses, or other syrup, with starches means fermentation. Soda will neutralize the resulting acids, it will not stop the fermentation.

For more than sixty years it has been the practice in *Hygienic* circles to take a large raw vegetable salad (leaving out tomatoes or other acid foods) with the starch meal. The salad has been a very large one, measured by ordinary standards and made up of fresh uncooked vegetables. This salad carries an abundance of vitamins and minerals. The vitamins in these vegetables are the genuine articles and no chemist's imitations of the real thing. No just-as-good substitutes for vitamins have ever satisfied *Hygienists*. We take the real article or nothing. Capsule-eating is a commercial program and belongs to the drug fetish.

Vitamins complement each other. We need, not just the vitamin B complex, but all vitamins. A large raw vegetable salad supplies several known vitamins and those that may exist but have not yet been detected. Vitamins not only cooperate with each other in the nutritive process, but they also cooperate with the minerals in the body. These are supplied by the vegetable salad. To take vitamin preparations that are combined with calcium or iron or other minerals will not answer the purpose. These minerals are in non-usable forms. There is no better source of food substances than the plant kingdom - the laboratory and the chemist have not yet been able to concoct acceptable foods.

Hygienists advise but one starch at a meal, not because there is any conflict in the digestion of these foods, but because taking two or more starches at a meal is practically certain to lead to overeating of this substance. We find it best, and this is doubly true in feeding the sick, to limit the starch intake to one starch at a meal. People with unusual powers of self-control may be permitted two starches, but these individuals are so rare, the rule should be: one *starch at a meal.*

The same author says: "Whether you eat hamburgers at the Greasy Spoon - or filet mignon at the Plaza - you're eating protein. Whether it's griddle cakes at the diner - or crepe suzette at the Astorbilt - you're eating carbohydrates. And whether it's oleomargarine from a relief agency, or butter balls at the Cafe de Lux - you're eating fat. These are the big three; the fourth part of food is roughage. All food will predominate in one of these substances or another. Some highly refined foods - like sugar - will contain only one of these, but - generally speaking, most foods contain all three - which is what makes the Hay Diet somewhat elusive."

It is not true that the fourth part of food is roughage, for roughage is not food, and it is not true that all foods predominate in one or the other of these four "parts of foods." Young, tender, growing plants have very little roughage, their cellulose being practically all digestible. They are valuable largely for their minerals and vitamins. His "big four" does not take into account the minerals that are in foods, and which are very abundant in many foods, while relatively scarce in others.

One may easily get the idea from reading the foregoing quotation, that one protein is as good as another, that one fat is as good as another, that any combination of food, such as hamburgers or filet mignon, is as good as any other, and that foods may be prepared in any manner desired. Its author is not actually guilty of holding any such views, but this statement of his could easily lead his readers to believe that just any old diet is good enough.

The remark that I wish to discuss is that, generally speaking, most foods contain carbohydrates, fats, proteins and roughage and that this makes the prohibition of protein-starch combinations "somewhat elusive." I want to differentiate between natural food combinations and the haphazard combinations commonly eaten. The human digestive tract is adapted to the digestion of natural combinations, but it is certainly not adapted to the digestion of the haphazard and indiscriminate combinations that are eaten in civilized life today. Natural combinations offer but little difficulty to the digestive system; but, it is one thing to eat one food, however complex its nature; it is quite another thing to eat two foods of "opposite character." The digestive juices may be readily adapted to one food, such as cereals, that is a protein-starch combination; they cannot be well adapted to two foods, such as bread and cheese. Tilden frequently said that nature never produced a sandwich.

It should be *axiomatic that our digestive system* is *adapted* to *the digestion of natural* combinations *and can handle the unnatural ones only with difficulty.* Modern civilized eating habits are so far removed from anything seen anywhere in nature or among so-called primitive peoples that it is impossible to think of them as being normal eating habits.

The prohibition is "somewhat elusive" to him simply because he has not given enough attention to the process of digestion. It is true that Nature puts up such combinations. It is true that these natural combinations offer but little difficulty to digestion. But, and here is the fact of digestion that all orthodox dietitians miss, the body is capable of so adapting its digestive secretions both as to strength of acid, concentration of enzymes and timing of secretions, to the digestive requirements of a particular food, while such precise adaptation of juices to foods is not possible when two different foods are eaten. The physiologist, Cannon, demonstrated that if starch is well mixed with saliva, it will continue to digest in the stomach for as much as two hours. This certainly cannot be true if proteins are eaten with the starch, for, in this case, the glands of the stomach will deluge the food with an acid gastric juice, thus rapidly ending gastric salivary digestion.

He says that the purpose of saliva is to begin the process of digestion of starches. "That is why", he adds, "you should chew bread, cereals, and other starchy foods very thoroughly; that is why you must not drink water through a mouthful of food. Though water at meal time is not condemned - it is needed to help the body in the chemistry of digestion - it must not be permitted to weaken the action of saliva on starches in the mouth."

The digestion of starches begins in the mouth, or should, but they remain in the mouth for such a short time that very little digestion takes place. Salivary digestion of starches can and will continue in the stomach for a long period if they are eaten under proper conditions. Eating acids and proteins with them will inhibit or completely suspend their digestion. Drinking water with the meal will weaken the action of saliva upon starches in the stomach as much as it will in the mouth, and it is not true that you need to drink at meal time to have water to aid in the digestion of your food. It will be best to drink your water ten to fifteen minutes before meals. If taken with meals it dilutes the digestive juices and then passes out of the stomach in short order carrying the digestive juices and their enzymes along with it.

The following menus constitute properly combined starch meals. It is suggested that the starch meal be eaten at noon time. Starches should be eaten dry and should be thoroughly chewed and insalivated before swallowing. Acids should not be eaten in the salad with the starch meal. We suggest a larger salad in the evening with the protein and a smaller one at noon with the starch. These menus may be eaten in amounts required by the individual.

Vegetable Salad	Vegetable Salad
Turnip Greens	Spinach
Yellow Squash	String Beans
Chestnuts	Coconut
Vegetable Salad	Vegetable Salad
String Beans	Spinach
Mashed Rutababa	Beets
Irish Potatoes	Irish Potatoes
Vegetable Salad	Vegetable Salad
String Beans	Asparagus
Turnips	White Squash
Sweet Potatoes	Yams
Vegetable Salad	Vegetable Salad
Beet Greens	Asparagus
Cauliflower	Okra
Sweet Potatoes	Peanuts

Vegetable Salad
Okra
Beet Greens
Whole Grain Bread

Vegetable Salad
String Beans
Yellow Squash
Irish Potatoes

Vegetable Salad
String Beans
Cabbage
Sweet Potatoes

Vegetable Salad
String Beans
Baked Egg Plant
Steamed Caladium Roots

Vegetable Salad
Kale
Okra
Jerusalem Artichokes

Vegetable Salad
Okra
String Beans
Jerusalem Artichokes

Vegetable Salad
Swiss Chard
Peas
Hubbard Squash

Vegetable Salad
Spinach
Cabbage
Baked Hubbard Squash

Vegetable Salad
Yellow Wax Beans
Kale
Irish Potatoes

Vegetable Salad
Okra
Brussels Sprouts
Irish Potatoes

Vegetable Salad
Spinach
Red Cabbage
Baked Caladium Roots

Vegetable Salad
Turnip Greens
Okra
Jerusalem Artichokes

Vegetable Salad
Spinach
Turnips
Jerusalem Artichokes

Vegetable Salad
Spinach
Cabbage
Chestnuts

Vegetable Salad
String Beans
Broccoli
Hubbard Squash

Vegetable Salad
Beet Greens
Yellow Squash
Irish Potatoes

Vegetable Salad
Kale
Okra
Brown Rice

Vegetable Salad
Beet Greens
Okra
Brown Rice

Vegetable Salad
Collards
Fresh Corn
Brown Rice

Vegetable Salad
Green Beans
Okra
Baked Hubbard Squash

Vegetable Salad
Green Peas
Carrots
Parsnips

Vegetable Salad
Spinach
Green String Beans
Brown Rice

Vegetable Salad
Chard
Asparagus
Baked Beans

Vegetable Salad
Okra
Beet Greens
Steamed Caladium Roots

Vegetable Salad
Spinach
Green Beans
Peanuts

Vegetable Salad
Turnip Greens
Asparagus
Brown Rice

Vegetable Salad
Beet Greens
Cauliflower
Baked Hubbard Squash

Vegetable Salad
Turnip Greens
Broccoli
Peanuts

Vegetable Salad
Chard
String Beans
Peanuts

Vegetable Salad
Chard
Okra
Brown Rice

Vegetable Salad
Swiss Chard
Yellow Squash
Baked Caladium Roots

EATING FRUITS

CHAPTER VII

William Henry Porter, M.D., says in his book, *Eating to Live Long,* that eating fruit "is one of the most pernicious and reprehensible of dietetic follies." But he admits that fruits eaten without other foods are alright. I doubt not that if he were approached on the subject of food combining, he would declare it to be a pernicious fad. Dr. Percy Howe of Harvard noted that people who could not eat oranges with meals were able to eat them alone without trouble. Dr. Dewey, of fasting fame, was strongly opposed to the eating of fruits, declaring that they demoralize digestion. None of these men knew anything of food combining. They merely noted that eating fruits with other foods results in a large amount of trouble, hence, they condemned, not the other foods, but the fruits. Actually, there is no more reason to condemn the fruit than there is to condemn the other food with which the fruit is taken.

Man, the archtype of the *cheirotheria,* should develop those frugivorous habits which are common to his anatomical structure, and from which he has largely departed in the course of time, due no doubt in large measure to his wanderings since he left his edenic home in the warmer regions. His sense of taste, being the expression of organic demand, must, of course, share in his health or his disease, and the taste which now demands flesh, will give place to a more exquisite appreciation of savors in the great varieties of fruits, vegetables and nuts in their many, varied and artistic combinations, which appeal as much to the eye and nose as to the tongue.

Fruits are among the finest and best of foods. Nothing affords us more good eating pleasure than a rich, mellow apple, a luscious, well-ripened banana, a carefully selected buttery, creamy, smooth avocado, or the wholesome, heart-warming goodness of a sweet grape. Real gustatory happiness is derived from the peach brought to the point of ripe perfection. Fruits, indeed, are a taste-enchanting, treasure trove of delightful eating enjoyment. With their luxury blends of rare flavors, delightful aromas, eye-pleasingcolors, fruits are always an invitation to pleasure in eating.

Fruits are more than just a delight to the eye, the nose and the mouth - they are master mixtures of pure, rich, real food elements. Few of them are rich in protein - the avocado and olive being the chief exceptions - but are packed full of mouth-watering sugars; are all-star flavor blends of acids, are full of minerals and vitamins. Together with nuts (which, botanically, are also classed as fruits) and green vegetables, fruits constitute an adequate diet - indeed, these foods constitute the ideal diet of the normally frugivorous animal: man.

Fruit eating affords us much deep-down pleasure. Mother Nature has flavored them just right to afford us the greatest enjoyment in eating. They are just right for our taste contentment. There is every reason why we should eat these foods with which Mother Nature so compellingly entices us to eating enjoyment and which she has filled with so much pure, rich, wholesome nourishment.

Nothing can afford us more gustatory happiness and real deep-down taste contentment than a meal of luscious fruits. Such a meal is always an invitation to pleasure. A fruit meal will not cause the troubles that flow from eating fruits with other foods. Such a meal will not demoralize digestion. It will do most for you. It is both refreshing and nourishing. The exquisite delight of eating such a naturally good meal, the wonderful feeling of comfort that follows, the real, genuine satisfaction it affords, far surpass that of eating other foods.

And this is the ideal manner in which to eat your fruits. Eat them at a fruit meal. The acids of fruits do not combine well with either starches or proteins; their sugars do not combine with either proteins or starches, the oils of the avocado and olive do not combine well with protein. Why risk digestive trouble by eating such foods with eggs, bread, etc.?[11]

Fruits undergo little or no digestion in the mouth and stomach and are, as a rule quickly sent into the intestine, where they undergo the little digestion they require. To eat them with other foods that do require considerable time in the stomach is to have them held up there pending the completion of the digestion of the other foods. Bacterial decomposition follows. We have previously considered this fact with reference to melons which are also fruits.

Fruits should not be eaten between meals. To eat them between meals is to put them into the stomach while the stomach is still busily engaged in digesting the previous meal. Trouble is sure to follow. Our rule, one from which we will do well not to vary, is to *eat fruit* at a *fruit meal.*

The habit of drinking quantities of fruit juices -lemon juice, orange juice, grapefruit juice, grape juice, tomato juice, papaya juice - between meals is responsible for a large amount of indigestion in those who think they are eating healthfully. This practice, revived during the last few years, was quite the vogue in *Hygienic* circles sixty to eighty years ago, and the digestive and other evils that flowed from it caused many to abandon the reform diet and return to their flesh pots. Let me recount Dr. Robert Walter's experience with the juice drinking fad, as he records it in his *Exact* Science *of Health.*

He says that in consequence of the treatments he had undergone in his efforts to recover health (first medical and then hydropathic), he had a "ravenous appetite for food" and as a consequence of the irritation of his stomach he had developed into a "gourmand which no amount of food could satisfy." He adds: "My sufferings from thirst were always great, but I did not like water, and having been taught the superior qualities of fruits, I could never get enough of the cooling juices, which fermented in my stomach, creating and perpetuating the very fever they temporarily relieved, all of which kept me in a fever of nervous hunger which no suffering in other respects ever equaled."

This experience caused the doctor to renounce vegetarianism and return to flesh eating. Eating at all hours of the day (for drinking juices is eating), he developed a neurosis which he mistook for hunger. Trying to satisfy a neurosis by eating is like trying to put out a fire with gasoline. Those who mistake gastric irritation for hunger and who continue to "appease" their "hunger" with the use of the cause of the irritation must grow from bad to worse. Turning from vegetarianism saved Dr. Walter, not because vegetarianism is wrong, but because he began to eat but one meal a day and ceased to imbibe fruit juices between meals.

No diet is so good but that it will be spoiled by the juice drinking practice and no diet is so bad but that this practice will make it worse. And this is true, not because the juices are bad, for they are excellent, but because their use in such manner disorganized digestion.

Many mistakes that are now being made by so-called dietitians could be avoided if they were acquainted with the history of diet reform. All of their "discoveries" were made and tried long ago, and some of those that are just now enjoying a heyday of popularity, were found evil and abandoned.

Although green vegetables form the ideal combination with nuts, acid fruits form a fair combination with these foods and may be taken with them. This, of course, has reference to protein nuts and not to the starch ones -coconuts, chestnuts, acorns, etc. Sweet fruits and nuts form a particularly objectionable combination, despite the delightful flavor of the mixture.

Avocados, containing more protein than milk, should not be combined with other proteins. Rich in fat, they also inhibit the digestion of other proteins. There can be no objection to combining them with acid fruits. They are best not eaten with sweet fruits. Nor should they be combined with nuts. In many quarters it is contended that the papaya assists in the digestion of proteins and we are strongly urged to eat it with proteins for this reason. Such a combination is not wise and, if it is true, as contended, that there is an enzyme in the papaya that will digest protein, it is an added reason not to combine it with protein. The employment of "aids to digestion" invariably weakens the health seeker's power of digestion. If his digestion is impaired, the sensible procedure is to remove the cause or causes of digestive impairment and then provide the digestive system with sufficient rest for repair and recuperation.

In feeding fruit meals to the sick, I have found it best to feed sweet fruits and the strongly acid fruits at separate meals. Thus, I do not feed dates or figs or bananas with oranges or grapefruit, or pineapples. Sugar, honey or other sweets with grapefruit is particularly objectionable. If your grapefruit is bitter or excessively sour, get the naturally superior grapefruit from the lower Rio Grande Valley of Texas.

The following menus constitute properly combined fruits and it is suggested that the fruit meal be eaten for breakfast. Do not add sugar to the fruits. Any fruit in season may be used. These meals may be eaten in amount required by the individual.

Oranges	Oranges
Grapefruit	Pineapple
Grapefruit	Papaya
Apples	Persimmons
Mangoes	Apples
Cherries	Grapes
Apricots	Figs
Fresh Figs	Cherries
Peaches	Apricots
Apricots	Plums
Bananas	Bananas
Pears	Persimmons
Grapes	Dates
Dates	Mangoes
Apples	Cherries
Pear	Apricots
Cherries	Berries with Cream
Peaches	(no sugar)
Nectarines	

Apples	Bananas
Grapes	Pear
Dates	Figs
Glass of Sour Milk	Glass of Sour Milk

As a variation, a very tasty meal may be made of a fruit salad and a protein as follows:

A large fruit salad composed of:
Grapefruit, Orange, Apple, Pineapple, Lettuce, Celery, Four ounces of Cottage Cheese or four ounces of nuts, or a greater amount of avocado.

In the Spring, a tasty salad may be made of the fruits in season:
Peach, Plum, Apricot, Cherry, Nectarine, Lettuce, Celery.

Sweet fruits - bananas, raisins, dates, figs, prunes, etc. - should not be put into the salad when it is intended to have a protein with it.

A SALAD A DAY
CHAPTER VIII

large raw vegetable salad with each dinner is one of the most important elements of the diet. As a preventive of disease, it is far superior to all the vaccines and serums ever devised. Salad eating, at least in this country, is a recent innovation and had its origin among those who have been dubbed food faddists. The addition of a suitable salad to a meal always improves the nutritional value of the meal.

At the turn of the century cooking was much worse than now and the diet was more gross - flesh, bread and potatoes or beans three times a day, with an assortment of side dishes, cakes, pies, etc., that would have made a meal for a 600 pound boar, all jumbled together in the most abominable combinations. It was an era when a flesh, bread and potato diet with such accessory foods as butter, cream, mayonnaise, sugar and sweet desserts were the most common reliance of the people. Fresh fruits and vegetables were scarce in the diet.

At that time the *medical* profession was horrified at the thought of eating uncooked fruits and vegetables. There were germs on them! "There are typhoid germs on all uncooked vegetables." But under the leadership of the "cranks," "faddists" and "quacks" the people took to eating these raw foods, and as the fresh foods entered the diet the germs vanished. No typhoid resulted from eating these germ-laden foods. Today, even the most bacteriophobic physicians eat these foods uncooked. The only food they refuse to eat without heat-sterilizing (it also contains typhoid and tubercular germs) is milk.

Although popular eating is less gross than formerly, people still overeat. They have relieved their stomachs and bowels to some extent but have thrown the burden on the liver, pancreas and ductless glands. Today the people are eating far more raw (uncooked) fruits and vegetables. Lettuce, cucumbers, celery, apples, strawberries, citrus fruits, etc., are raised in enormous quantities and shipped by train-loads to all parts of the country. Train-loads of lettuce are now raised where wheelbarrow-loads were formerly raised.

Until well within the lifetime of the author the *medical* profession advised never to eat "raw" fruits and vegetables because of the germs they carried. Not until it was discovered that raw fruits and vegetables were the best sources of vitamins (and this discovery came only after the profession was forced to recognize that people were getting well on diets of uncooked fruits and vegetables) did they cease to warn against the germ-laden uncooked fruits and vegetables.

Indeed, they are still issuing the old warning when one goes into Mexico, India, China and elsewhere.

Nature turns out her products in a state of physiological balance and when we eat our foods as she produces them, they are not sources of trouble. But when we extract portions of her products, as when sugar is extracted from cane or beet or white flour is extracted from wheat, we eat an artificial product that is out of balance, lacking in many of the essentials of nutrition. The remedy for such a state of affairs is to eat whole, that is, unprocessed, unrefined and uncooked foods grown on fertile soil.

A salad of uncooked, non-starchy vegetables should accompany every protein and every starch meal. The common practice of eating shrimp salad, potato salad and similar salads will not suffice.[12] Indeed, such dishes hardly merit the name salad. The salad should consist of such foods as lettuce, celery, cucumbers, green and red peppers (the non-pungent varieties of peppers), cabbage, tomatoes and other non-starchy vegetables. These foods should be served fresh and without salt, vinegar, olive oil, mayonnaise or dressings of any kind. Tomatoes should form part of the salad only when proteins are eaten and not when starches are taken at the meal. Such foods as onions, garlic, water cress, radishes and bitter foods are not recommended for salads nor to be eaten in any other way.

To assure a plentiful supply of minerals and vitamins, a large salad, as suggested above, should accompany each protein and each carbohydrate meal. The customary salad consisting of two leaves of wilted lettuce and a slice of half-ripe tomato, topped off with a radish or pickled olive and a spoonful of greasy foul tasting salad dressing, is not only unwholesome but does not meet the vitamin and mineral needs of a canary. A salad should be part of the most enjoyable food of a meal and will be if proper choices of salad materials are made.

I coined the slogan "a salad a day keeps acidosis away." It is true, however, only if the salad is of the right kind. Shrimp salad, potato salad, egg salad and salad covered with oil or vinegar will not answer the purpose assigned to salads.

The word salad is from a Latin word meaning salt, and our salad vegetables are abundant sources of mineral salts in their most readily assimilated form. There is no substitute for green foods in our diet. It is important that these be taken, largely if not wholly, in the raw or uncooked state. In general, the green leaves of plants are our richest sources of organic salts (minerals), are rich sources of vitamins, are sources of small quantities of the highest grade proteins and are the best sources of chlorophyl, which, while it will not deodorize your breath and body, is essential in animal nutrition.

Salads are not so important in the diet of one who lives largely on uncooked foods and whose diet is made up largely of fruits and vegetables. One who eats largely of flesh, cereals, legumes and other starchy and high protein foods has an urgent need for one or two large green salads daily.

A British author says that "two or three hundred years ago our meat-gorging ancestors, if they happened to be wealthy enough to gorge on meat, went through a fifteen course meal without the mention of fruit, from duck to chicken, to pork and pheasant, then fish and meat again, till they gasped and often passed out in surfeit or apoplexy. Some Red Indian tribes, living almost entirely on meat, scorned fruit and vegetables as woman's food, and the hunters of Asia and Africa, though there are really only a few of them, do not make much fuss over fruit." Taking a salad with a meal of that kind is somewhat on the order of taking an antidote with a poison.

Of the number of green foods that are commonly eaten in this country, the following is not a complete list, but contains a sufficient number to show the variety of foods that we use: spinach, kale, chard, turnip greens, beet greens, cabbage, broccoli, okra, green beans, fresh peas, asparagus, collards, lettuce, celery, Chinese cabbage, Bok choy, etc. All of these vegetables are palatable in the raw state and may profitably be added to a salad. There are several varieties of lettuce that may be used, often two or more kinds at a time. In some parts of the nation escarole, endive and other green vegetables are obtainable. The cucumber makes a very delightful addition to a salad and may be eaten whole.

The variety of different salads that may be made is great and one or more of these may be had at all seasons of the year. Indeed, it is important to have some fresh green food every day of the year and not take salads only at intervals. It is well to eat a large salad and not skimp on this part of the meal. The salads served in most homes, restaurants, cafeterias, hotels and other eating places are commonly too small to adequately meet the needs of the persons eating them. A big salad should always be the rule.

I get complaints from many people that they cannot take so much of what they call "roughage." Dr. Kellogg pointed out years ago that this so-called "roughage" (fiber) was better termed "bulk." The fact is that the small amount of indigestible cellulose in these foods is not rough. It is, on the contrary, rather soft and filled with water. On the other hand, if a large salad is run through a juice extractor and all the water extracted from it, it will be seen at once that the amount of bulk in what looks like an enormous salad is but a small measure. The cry that they contain too much "roughage" is not based on fact. When vegetables and fruits are sliced, cut small, ground, shredded, or otherwise broken into small particles, so that the oxygen of the air gets to them, much food value is lost through oxidation. The longer they are permitted to stand before eating, after they have been thus treated, the greater is the loss of food value. The loss of certain vitamins through oxidation is especially rapid. Such practices are permissible only when feeding the toothless individual who is unable to chew whole foods. Then the food should be fed immediately after preparing, so that a minimum of loss through oxidation is sustained.

The dressings added to salads are not incompatible with the salads per se, but they do interfere with the digestion of other foods. Acids used in the dressings interfere with the digestion of both starches and proteins. Oils added to the salad interfere with the digestion of proteins. Whether cream is sweet or sour, its addition to the salad will interfere with protein digestion. Sugar added to the salad dressing inhibits protein digestion. Thus, while there is no serious reason why oil or cream may not be added to a salad when it is to be taken with a starch meal; it should not be added to a salad that is to be taken with a protein meal. Lemon juice and vinegar should not be added with either meal. There can be no objection to the addition of lemon juice or oil or both to the salad if a salad is to be taken alone as we often like to do, or as often happens, the salad and a cooked green vegetable is to be eaten as the meal.

Tomato acid interferes with the digestion both of protein and starch. Thus it is wise to omit tomatoes from the salad when either of these types of foods are to be eaten. In the cases of cheese, nuts and avocado, all three of which contain oils which inhibit protein digestion longer than the acid of the starch will do so, there is no reason why tomatoes may not be eaten with these protein foods. When these foods are taken, perhaps there can be no serious objection to the use of lemon juice or oil on the salad. With other proteins, follow the rule to *eat acids and proteins at separate meals.*

On the whole, I prefer the plain undressed salad made of whole vegetables without all of the customary shredding and chopping. Rather than slice the tomatoes that go into the salad, place a whole tomato in the middle of the salad and build around it for an artistic effect. The vitamin C in tomatoes is rapidly destroyed by oxidation when these are cut into thin slices. An equally rapid loss of vitamin C takes place in lettuce when this is cut up into small pieces. If leaf lettuce, such as romaine lettuce is used, serve the leaves whole. If head lettuce is used, cut the heads in half or in quarters, depending upon their size. A large amount of lettuce should be served with the salad. If cucumbers are added to the salad, serve them whole if they are small, or cut in half if they are large. The smaller cucumbers are most tasty and are not bitter. Serve celery stalks whole, rather than grated or cut into small pieces. Carrots should not be grated.

Salads are best made simple. Complex salads made of half a dozen to a dozen ingredients are far from ideal. Three to four articles of food in a salad are sufficient. Lettuce, tomatoes and celery make an excellent salad. If to this you want to add a sprig of parsley or a piece of red bell pepper for color and flavor, this may be done. Celery, lettuce and cucumber make an excellent salad. Romaine lettuce, young, tender okra, and spinach make a tasty and satisfying salad. Cabbage, tomato and young, fresh peas also make a tasty and satisfying salad. In fact, there is almost no end to the variety and combinations of salads that may be made, each packed with an abundance of much needed minerals and vitamins.

It is vitally important that growing children have a daily salad. Indeed, the salad is more important for the growing child than for the adult, although it is very important for the adult. Children should be started early in life with their daily salad so that they build a keen relish for it and continue to eat it for the rest of their lives. This will be found to be far more satisfactory in the diet of the child than any preparation that may be purchased from the drug store, such as cod liver oil, minerals and vitamin concentrates, etc. These salads are more acceptable sources of calcium than is milk and this is doubly so now that it is almost impossible to get anything other than pasteurized milk. It cannot be emphasized too often or too strongly that pasteurization alters the calcium salts in milk so that they are no longer of use to the child. Let me end this chapter by saying *there* is no *substitute for the* green *foods* in *our diet.*

EATING SCHEDULE
FOR A WEEK

Ail the menus given in this book are intended merely as guides to the reader to assist him in understanding the principles of food combining and to enable him to work out his own menus. It is my thought that it is more important to know how to make up one's own menus than to have a book of menus giving three meals a day for every day in the year. The person who understands food combining and who is able to arrange his own menus is never at a loss, wherever he is, in preparing his meals. He can devise a meal from the foods at hand.

The same foods are not always available in all parts of the country. A food that is available in one section of the country at one time of the year may be available in another part of the country at a different time of the year. Food availability varies with season, climate, altitude, soil and market facilities. The man who knows how to combine his meals may make use of the foods that are at hand and work out a meal. The man who depends on a cut and dried book of menus and does not know how to combine his foods may find that the particular foods listed in the menu for today are not available - he is left out on a limb. What he usually does is take the easy way and eat indiscriminately. If you are at the home of a friend or relative, your book of menus can be of no service to you; but if you know how to combine your foods, you may usually pick out compatible combinations from the foods spread before you and eat a well-combined meal.

Learn the principles of food combining so that you may properly apply them in any and all circumstances in which you may find yourself. A child may be able to follow a chart; an intelligent adult should learn principles and learn to apply these. Once you have done this and have practiced properly combining your foods for a time, the practice becomes automatic and you do not have to spend a lot of time on it. Above all things, do not become a crank on the matter. Eat your meal and forget it. Let your friends eat their foods and don't give them a lecture on dietetics at the dining table.

The following two weekly schedules are designed to demonstrate the proper ways to combine foods at different seasons of the year. The first week's schedule covers foods available in Spring and Summer. The second week's schedule covers foods available in Fall and Winter. Use these merely as guides and learn to prepare your own menus.

BREAKFAST	LUNCH	DINNER
SUNDAY		
Watermelon	Vegetable Salad Chard Yellow Squash Potatoes	Vegetable Salad String Beans Okra Nuts
MONDAY		
Peaches Cherries Apricots	Vegetable Salad Beet Greens Carrots Baked Beans	Vegetable Salad Spinach Cabbage Cottage Cheese
TUESDAY		
Cantaloupes	Vegetable Salad Okra Green Squash Jerusalem Artichokes	Vegetable Salad Broccoli Fresh Corn Avocado
WEDNESDAY		
Berries with Cream *(no sugar)*	Vegetable Salad Cauliflower Okra Brown Rice	Vegetable Salad Green Squash Turnip Greens Soy Sprouts[13]
THURSDAY		
Nectarines Apricots Plums	Vegetable Salad Green Cabbage Carrots Sweet Potatoes	Vegetable Salad Beet Greens String Beans Nuts
FRIDAY		
Watermelon	Vegetable Salad Baked Eggplant Chard Whole Wheat Bread	Vegetable Salad Yellow Squash Spinach Eggs
SATURDAY		
Bananas Cherries Glass of Sour Milk	Vegetable Salad Green Beans Okra Irish Potatoes	Vegetable Salad Kale Broccoli Soy Sprouts

BREAKFAST	*LUNCH*	*DINNER*
SUNDAY		
Grapes	Vegetable Salad	Vegetable Salad
Bananas	Chinese Cabbage	Spinach
Dates	Asparagus	Yellow Squash
	Baked Caladium Roots	Baked Beans
MONDAY		
Persimmons	Vegetable Salad	Vegetable Salad
Pear	Kale	Brussels Sprouts
Grapes	Cauliflower	String Beans
	Yams	Pecans
TUESDAY		
Apples	Vegetable Salad	Vegetable Salad
Grapes	Turnip Greens	Kale
Dried Figs	Okra	Yellow Squash
	Brown Rice	Avocado
WEDNESDAY		
Pears	Vegetable Salad	Vegetable Salad
Persimmons	Broccoli	Okra
Banana	String Beans	Spinach
Glass of Sour Milk	Irish Potatoes	Pignolias
THURSDAY		
Papaya	Vegetable Salad	Vegetable Salad
Orange	Carrots	Chard
	Spinach	Yellow Squash
	Steamed Caladium Roots	Unprocessed Cheese
FRIDAY		
Persimmons	Vegetable Salad	Vegetable Salad
Grapes	Green Squash	Red Cabbage
Dates	Parsnips	String Beans
	Whole Grain Bread	Sunflower Seeds
SATURDAY		
Grapefruit	Vegetable Salad	Vegetable Salad
	Fresh Peas	Spinach
	Kale	Steamed Onions
	Coconut	Baked Beans[14]

REMEDYING INDIGESTION

I t is impossible to overestimate the importance of good digestion. Upon the efficiency of the digestive process depends the preparation of the raw materials of nutrition; hence, upon good digestion depends, to a very large extent, the well-being of the body. There can be no such thing as good nutrition without good digestion. The best of diets fails to yield up its greatest good when the digestive process fails in the work of preparing it for use by the body.

Poor digestion cannot be depended upon to supply the materials' with which to build and maintain good blood; hence the tissues will be inadequately nourished, the general health must fail and the constitution deteriorate. It is of great importance to remember that the normal process of blood making depends upon the first step in the preparation of blood-making materials in the digestive tract. Good digestion, therefore, means more normal tissue change throughout the body. Improved digestion results in general improvement in all of the functions of life. Many and great are the benefits to flow from improved digestion.

Indigestion is the forerunner, not the cause, of many of man's more serious ills. But every impairment of function becomes a secondary source of cause, and the poisoning and starvation that result from indigestion are added causes of suffering. These are superadded to the primary causes of man's suffering. When indigestion is prevented, health is preserved; when it is remedied, health is restored.

A whole train of discomforts or symptoms accompany the progressive impairment of the function of digestion, such as gas, sour eructations, a sense of discomfort running into pain in the abdomen, sleepless and unrefreshing nights, furred tongue in the morning, absence of desire for food, constipation, foul stools, nervousness, etc. This is by no means an exhaustive catalogue of the symptoms that accompany indigestion.

If we reflect for a minute upon the enormous quantities of baking soda (bicarbonate of soda), Milk of Magnesia, Alka-Seltzer, Bromo-Seltzer, Tums, Bellans, charcoal, and other drugs that are daily consumed by the American people to relieve them of distress arising out of acid fermentation and gas in the digestive tract, all of this growing out of indigestion, we may readily reach the conclusion that, as a people, we are suffering from indigestion. Distress after meals is exceedingly common and nobody seems to know how to do more than give the sufferers a few minutes to a few hours of respite from their distress. It is a sad commentary upon the much touted "science" of medicine that it can do nothing lasting or constructive in a simple functional condition of this nature.

Besides the drugs employed to temporarily allay distress, there are many "aids to digestion" in use. Pepsin is, perhaps, the best known of these. For a time, chewing gum was declared to aid the digestion of food. These "aids to digestion" are all frauds. They do not aid digestion at all. They do not in any way improve or increase the functioning powers of the digestive organs and they do not remove any of the causes of digestive impairment. On the contrary, the continued use of anyone of them or all of them, without exception, further impairs the digestive powers.

The use of "digestive aids" and of means to "relieve" distress keeps the attention of the users directed away from the true solution of their problems and prevents them from learning the truth about their health and disease and how they may truly recover the former. That mankind has so long relied upon such measures, which have always failed, is a constant source of amazement to me. One expects even fools to learn from repeated experiences.

A view frequently expressed by medical authors and apparently held by the whole profession, is that if two foods may be digested *separately,* they may be digested together. They extend this principle to cover the whole menu: if each article of food in the bill-of-fare is separately digestible, then they are digestible if eaten in a twenty-one course dinner, the diner partaking of everything from soup to nuts.

In a limited way, this view is true, else would conventional eaters die from lack of food. Instead of dying, they thrive after a fashion, many of them even growing fat on the conventional diet with its haphazard mixtures. That digestion is not very efficient, as shown, however, by gas, sour eructations, discomforts, foul stools and the presence of large quantities of undigested food in the stools. At least half of the food eaten by most people is passed out undigested.

It is commonly held that food may be taken into the digestive tract in the most indiscriminate and haphazard manner, in any possible combination, and in whatever amount the eater may desire and they will be well and efficiently digested. This view is not based upon physiology, but upon the determination of the profession that the customary practices of the people shall not be disturbed. Every student of physiology is well aware that the digestive enzymes have certain well-defined limitations and that different digestive juices are secreted for use in digesting different kinds of food substances. These limitations should be respected in our eating habits.

The fact is that millions of Americans do eat in the indiscriminate and haphazard manner that the medical profession endorses and suffer with indigestion after every meal. The millions in profits that are made yearly out of the sale of Alka-Seltzer, Bellans, Rolaids, Pepto-Bismol, Lacto Bismadine and similar drugs prescribed by physicians, while many people continue to rely upon baking soda for relief from their distress, signifies nothing. Perhaps, as the profession contends, digestion is efficient. Or does it simply mean that to provide the people with a simple means of avoiding all of this distress will cut in sharply on profits and fees?

To the objection of taking milk with flesh they point out that people regularly cook milk with certain flesh foods, such as crabs, oysters, etc., and do not die of acute poisoning. The idea here expressed is simply that if a thing is customarily done, it must be good. Man has never adopted and continued a harmful custom - not in all history. The only sane thing for any man to do is to eat, drink and smoke and give no attention to his health until he has lost it, and then go to a physician for a pill or a shot in the arm. If the people are in the habit of taking milk and flesh at the same meal, this custom should not be discontinued, no matter how much evidence there may be that it is a hurtful practice.

That haphazard eaters may learn to combine their foods by rules that are based on the physiology of digestion and escape the indigestion, foul stools, gas and discomfort that accompany conventional eating, is a fact that any doubter may discover for himself by giving the matter a fair test. Any medical man who will give it a test may discover this for himself. That medical men pretend that they are "scientific" and are wedded to the "scientific method" while refusing to put the matter to a test is an evidence of their prejudice and bigotry. They reject the "scientific method" if and when there is reason to think that the results of a test may disturb the customs of the people and practices of the profession. The test might show them to be wrong.

Any student of the eating practices of mankind knows well that the eating practices of present day Americans are very modern and that the indiscriminate jumbling together of all kinds of food in the stomach has not been practiced by mankind in the past. The further back we go in our study of man's eating practices, the simpler we find them. We know, also, as a matter of present -day experience, that simple eating provides for better digestion. When we view the eating habits of the animals below us, we find the utmost simplicity. In general, in fact, they tend to eat but one food at a meal. It would probably be impossible to induce an ape, for example, to eat a seven course dinner, much less could he be induced to eat a twenty-one course meal.

We are faced today with two concomitant facts that may be shown to be related to each other as cause and effect. We have, as fact number one, the haphazard and indiscriminate mixing of a great variety of foods at one meal. We have, as fact number two, tile almost universal indigestion, accompanied by the taking of drugs to relieve the resulting discomfort. Now if it can be shown that simple meals are easily digested and rarely give rise to indigestion, while the complex mixtures regularly eaten are followed by almost universal indigestion, we are faced with a group of facts that are not to be ignored.

The old adage has it that "the proof of the pudding is in the eating thereof." I would suggest to my readers that the proof of the value of properly combining foods is in the eating of combinations that conform to the rules we have formulated. If such meals end the indigestion, there may be more in the practice than its foes are willing to admit. Certainly food combinations that do not result in indigestion are preferable to indiscriminate eating accompanied with indigestion. Certainly it is better to digest the food well than to take drugs, which also interfere with the digestion of food. Drugs provide a temporary respite from the discomforts of indigestion, but they encourage the very style of eating that results in indigestion besides producing evils of their own.

"There are none so blind as those who can see and won't," runs an old adage. Intelligent people who close their eyes to the facts of physiology and those of experience in food combining that is based on the facts of digestion, not only blind themselves but guarantee themselves much needless discomfort and suffering.

It is obvious to every intelligent reader of this book that a radically different approach to this subject is required if we are to successfully remedy indigestion. We gain nothing but added disease by enriching the manufacturers and distributors of drugs. These make millions out of substances that only add to the suffering of the poor deluded victims of the drug fetish. *Natural Hygiene* offers the people a real escape from their suffering and their bondage to ancient fallacies.

Good digestion is normal and when indigestion is present, it means that the powers of life have been reduced, usually by the conduct of the individual so suffering. After making due allowance for the effects of an unfavorable environment, we must ascribe most of the sufferings of men and women to the evil, though ignorant it may be, and systematic departure from organic laws in the general mode of life. The state of health is only to be maintained by a due observance of all the laws of life in their combination.

How much more efficient is the process of digestion when food is taken in a serene and unexcited state of mind, compared with the working of the same process when food is taken in a state of mental agitation, from whatever source derived! And how greatly is the process of digestion affected by the conduct of the same person after meals, in relation to repose or work! Rest after eating is indispensable to good digestion. No man can digest his food well who only half masticates it and who bolts from his dining table to his business like a greyhound slipped from the leash.

When life is lived at such a pace, as it often is in the larger cities, that everything, including eating, is done at breathless speed, when the jaws cannot masticate fast enough, and the food is gulped down half chewed, when the "eater" rushes immediately back to work without any rest whatever of body or mind, and this from day to day and from year to year, so long as the powers of life hold out, the Nemesis of outraged nature takes its toll. No man's capacity for continuing a galley-slave life is limitless, but capacity varies depending upon variations in the constitutional powers of different individuals. The stronger will hold out longer than his weaker brother, but sooner or later the most robust must succumb to the exhausting effects of such a life.

Whether through want or redundancy, through dissipation or overexertion of any kind, when the human constitution becomes impaired and vitality fails, one of the first symptoms of the vital depression is an enfeeblement of the powers of digestion.

We have only to consider for a moment the many influences that certainly lessen the bodily vigor of man to realize that everybody in civilized society is more or less enervated. We may divide these influences roughly into sins of commission and sins of omission. Sins of omission may be said to be the offspring of ignorance of the laws of life or of willful neglect, or both. Sins of commission are those where the laws of life are not only wittingly neglected, but where they are positively and of purpose violated in the pursuit of either business or of pleasure. The same enervating influences may, perhaps, also be divided into those which are forced upon mankind by the necessities and struggles of life (by a socio-economic environment over which he, as an individual, has no control), and those which are adventitious, or in a manner, self-sought. The evils of the misery and poverty of the poorer classes are matched by those of the dissipations and enervating luxuries of the wealthy classes. Speculation, gambling and excitements of every kind make the largest drains on the nervous system. However, and from whence arising, whether from unavoidable over-toil of the mental and physical worker, or from the suicidal indulgence of the man of fashion, or from a combination of both these broad factors, the result is the same.

With the habitual violation of the laws of life, or more narrowly, with the habitual indulgence in enervating activities, the slow sapping of the energies of the constitution results in a progressive enervating of the body - a state of lowered nerve energy not always recognized at first and the warnings not readily listened to - but as sure in its downward progress as the loosened avalanche. The result is the prostration of the bodily and mental powers and the degradation of the whole man.

Whenever, through a continual violation of the laws of life, the constitutional powers become enfeebled, not only is the excretory function greatly weakened, giving rise to toxemia (a state of poisoning by the retention of normal body waste), but also the digestive and assimilative powers become impoverished so that the nutrition of the body is lowered commensurate with the degree of constitutional enfeeblement. Indigestion follows with its consequent slow starving of the sufferer.

In such an enfeebled individual no change of diet can bring about a restoration of health until after all the causes of general enervation have been removed and sufficient rest has been secured to enable the body to restore its functioning activities. It should be obvious that if the power to digest and assimilate food is not increased, all attempts to "build-up" the health seeker by any kind of feeding program will prove abortive and useless. It is even more futile to attempt to restore digestive power by the use of drugs - tonics, astringents, barks, mineral acids, preparations of iron, etc. - as these only further impair an already greatly impaired constitution and add to the digestive enfeeblement.

To substitute one source of enervation for another is not a rational procedure. To undertake to rest, while, at the same time, undergoing a whole series of palliating treatments - baths, massages, electrical treatments, adjustments, colonic irrigations, enemas, etc., - is to fail to achieve full health. Bear in mind that when you learn to live in conformity with the laws of life you will be forever delivered from the torture of the futile effort to destroy the necessary consequences of your misconduct. Only when we have learned to live within the confines of physiological and biological law can we transmute into a song of gladness that moan of pain and wail of despair that goes up from the earth today.

The intelligent person, viewing the great number of so-called diseases that arise out of this prostration of the functions of life, and realizing that they have one and all grown out of the habitual violations of the laws of life, will recognize at once that the first step in the restoration of health needs must be to make amends at once by an unconditional return to simplicity and perfect obedience to the laws that have been so perseveringly violated. The health seeker, it should be evident, must be brought back to that completely healthful manner of life from which, alone, in its totality, we know that there is prospect of effecting a genuine restoration of health.

Is it possible to imagine a health seeker being rationally treated after a different manner? Can we conceive of a health seeker, while adhering steadfastly in his manner of life, to the identical habits which gave rise to his suffering, to be cured by drugs, or serums, or vaccines, or by surgery? Plainly it is impossible, unless, of course, we cast our physiology and, along with it, our common sense, to the four winds.

In the first place, the health seeker's nervous system having been prostrated from overwork, over indulgence, stimulation (irritation), and excesses of many and varied kinds, it is plain that he must, above all things, have rest. Accordingly, we would order a pre-emptory release from all mental and bodily activities and duties that constitute a drain upon his energy resources. This is the *sine que none* of recovery. It is plain that, above all things, the enervated individual must have rest and this must include mental repose as well as bodily rest.

The physiological importance of repose of the mind to the performance of the function of digestion, on the healthy performance of which, as previously stated, vital results depend, explains the overriding importance which we have attached to the principles of nervous repose. Mental rest is best secured, by a change of scenes from the haunts of business or pleasure, in the gas-laden atmosphere of the towns and cities, with their incessant noise and hubbub, to the delights of a quiet country retreat in some picturesque district abounding in pleasant and varied scenery, with fresh breezes of health to play about the health seeker arid over-head from morning to night, where he may enjoy the quiet repose of nature and bask in her healthful sunshine.

These subjects discover that, in the long run, drugs do not answer the needs of their problem. On the contrary, they find themselves growing daily worse while resorting to drugs and resort to larger and larger doses, or to frequent changes of drugs. This progressive deterioration of function is due not alone to the impairing effects of the drugs, but also to the neglect of the original impairing causes, which the resort to drugs guarantees. It is hopeless to think of *curing* a disease while the manner of life that is the radical cause of all the trouble is persevered in.

The "two paths" of life are open to all alike. One leads to health, strength, happiness and longer life. It crowns us with honor and gives us a richer, fuller, more abundant life. The other leads as surely to disease, weakness, unhappiness and premature death as the cast stone falls back to earth. It crowns us with dishonor and gives us pains and an empty life. Which path will you follow? The choice is yours; nor can anyone else make the choice for you. Law and order are not respectors of persons and everyone will be rewarded or penalized according to the life he lives.

Are you dissipating or spending time and money on an abnormal appetite? What are your habits? Are they lawful (physiological) and such as you can expect good to flow from? Are you indulging in games of chance or in perverted practices? Are you certain that your mode of living - your mental and physical practices - conform with the laws of life? Keep in mind always that it is the right use of the body and mind that provides for man the best development and highest happiness.

Nor, can we approach the problem before us with any single-factor solution. We are dealing with a state of affairs that has grown out of a varied assortment of antecedent factors and it can be remedied only by duly considering each of these elemental causative factors. It is not enough to enjoin one enervating habit. All must be stopped at once and refrained from thereafter, if true success is to crown our efforts.

Just as the first step in the restoration of functioning power to the enfeebled organism is the discontinuance of all enfeebling practices, so the second step in the restoration of power to the enervated constitution is rational use of the combined materials and influences that constitute the *Hygienic System.* After all causes of enfeeblement have been removed, rest, sleep, food of the proper kind, exercise, fresh air, pure water, sunshine and healthful mental and moral influences are essential to the restortion of integrity of structure and efficiency of function.

When once, by *Hygienic* means, the body has been freed of its load of toxins, its nerve energy has been restored to normal. Elimination has been reestablished and the digestive and assimilative powers have been restored, there follows a gradual return to health. Until this has been done, the best of diets will not and cannot give the desired results. How many health seekers have sunk into their graves, in chronic as well as in acute disease, amid the strictest regulations of their diets, thus attesting the inefficacy of diet to preserve the sick and restore them to health, when disconnected from the series of appropriate *Hygienic* materials and influences.

Hygienic factors are not of great importance in local treatment, but have their greatest, or sole value in their benefits to the whole organism. Thus, while food is of no value when applied locally, its value when used by the whole body, is undisputed. Hence, as an indispensable basis of the work of the *Hygienist,* we must endeavor to secure to the health seeker the full benefit of all the *Hygienic* means, in their entire plentitude, for only thus can the health seeker be given a fair chance of recovery. Thus understood, the phrase *Natural Hygiene* acquires a real significance, at once novel, startling, intense and delicious.

It is necessary to emphasize that food alone, important as it is in both health and disease, is not enough to assure either the preservation or the restoration of health. It is only in its physiological connection with water, exercise, rest, sleep and other elements of the *Hygienic System* that its true value becomes manifest. Of these combined means, contributing severally to the remedial processes of the body, and each essential to these processes, it is enough to point out that it would be impossible to assign superior value to any over the rest, the simple fact being that each is indispensable, and that health is restored under the *Hygienic System* not by one *Hygienic* factor alone, but through the combined remedial use of all of them.

It cannot be too strongly insisted upon, as a scientific fact, that it is the whole of the aforementioned *Hygienic* factors, in their plenary combination and harmonious co adaptation to the physiological wants of the living organism, which consitute the material and subtle means employed by the organism in the restoration of health. The natural or *Hygienic* care of the sick, made up, as it is, of so many concurrent and interdependent factors, cannot be held responsible for the failures that attend the unscientific and wholly one-sided application of some one or two *Hygienic* elements by the ignorant and inexperienced.

Physiological rest - fasting - is of value in all forms of impaired health, but in indigestion it is a sure means of providing rest for an overworked digestive system. In fasting practically all of the organs of the body reduce their activities, hence they rest. The exceptions are the organs of elimination (excretion) and these step up their activities: hence, during the fast the body is enabled to free itself of its accumulated load of toxic waste. The combination of mental, physical and physiological rest constitutes an ideal means of promoting elimination.

The fast should not be undertaken at home, where there are distractions, annoyances, and responsibilities and where friends and relatives interpose objections to it. It is best taken in a Hygienic institution under the supervision of an experienced Hygienist. In the Hygienic institution the health seeker is in a position, both physically and mentally, that makes it comparatively easy, not only to fast, but also to break bad habits. Here, too, is the place for him to cultivate and fix new and good habits. Indeed, it will always be best for the health seeker to remain in the institution until the new habits have become so much a part of him that he will experience little difficulty in continuing them once he has returned home. This is vitally important to continued progress in health and in preserving health, once this has been regained.

Let us not close our eyes to the obvious fact that health, when lost, can only be re-acquired by a laborious process in which the health seeker himself must play, by far, the principal role, and must faithfully and manfully carry out that fundamental truth in a systematic routine of healthful practices, till the end is achieved.

NOTES

Original wording from the previous printings of *Food Combining Made Easy*

1. As this book has been prepared for the general reader and not for the vegetarian only, the menus contained herein include meals for the mixed-diet eater as well as meals for the vegetarian. This has not been done as a matter of compromise, nor yet as a tacit desertion of vegetarianism, but as a means of meeting the requirements of all classes of readers.

2. When the average man or woman eats flesh, or eggs, or cheese, he or she takes bread with the protein. Hot-dogs, ham sandwiches, hamburgers, toast and eggs, ham on rye, and similar combinations of protein and starch represent the common practice of eating such foods.

3. When one eats a hamburger or a hot dog, one does not eat his flesh first and then follow with his bun.

4. By this is meant that cereals, bread, potatoes and other starch foods, should be eaten separately from flesh, eggs, cheese, nuts and other protein foods.

5. It is logical, therefore, to assume that eggs should not be taken with flesh or milk.

6. This may not mean that two different kinds of flesh may not be taken together or that two different kinds of nuts may not be taken at the same time; but it certainly means that such protein combinations as flesh and eggs, flesh and nuts, flesh and cheese, eggs and milk, eggs and nuts, cheese and nuts, milk and nuts, etc., should not be taken.

7. In other words, such foods as cream, butter, oils of various kinds, gravies, fat meats, etc., should not be consumed at the same meal with nuts, cheese, eggs, flesh.

8. (removed) Vegetable Salad
   Chard
   Yellow Squash
   Lamb Chops

9. (removed) Vegetable Salad
   Green Squash
   Turnip Greens
   Roast Beef

10. (removed) Vegetable Salad
    String Beans
    Okra
    Broiled Lamb

11. Why risk digestive trouble by eating such foods with flesh, eggs, bread, etc.?

12. The common practice of eating shrimp salad, potato salad and similar salads will not suffice.

13. (This particular menu originally called for lamb chops.)

14. (This particular menu originally called for lamb chops.)

Book Publishing Co.

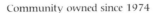

Community owned since 1974

books that educate, inspire, and empower

To find your favorite vegetarian and soyfood products online, visit:
www.healthy-eating.com

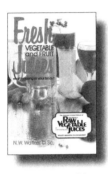

Fresh Vegetable
and Fruit Juices
Norman W. Walker, DSc
978-0-89019-033-3
$9.95

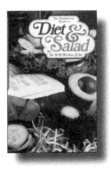

Diet & Salad
Norman W. Walker, DSc
978-0-89019-034-0
$9.95

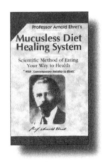

Mucusless Diet
Healing System
Professor Arnold Ehret
978-1-884772-00-9
$4.95

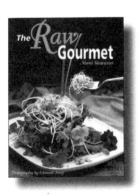

The Raw Gourmet
Nomi Shannon
978-0-92047-048-0
$24.95

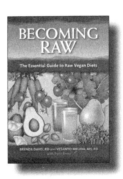

Becoming Raw
Brenda Davis, RD,
Vesanto Melina, MS, RD,
with Rynn Berry
978-1-57067-238-5
$24.95

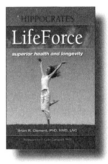

Hippocrates LifeForce
Brian R. Clement, PhD, NMD, LNC
978-1-57067-249-1
$14.95

Purchase these health titles and cookbooks from your local bookstore or natural food store,
or you can buy them directly from:

Book Publishing Company • P.O. Box 99 • Summertown, TN 38483 • 1-800-695-2241

Please include $3.95 per book for shipping and handling.